PHYSICIAN UNLEASHED:
The Physician Freedom Formula

A Roadmap to Help More People, Earn More Money and Live the Life of Your Dreams

By Tamika Henry, MD, MBA
and Malaika Woods, MD, MPH

Publisher: The Abundant Physician, 4963 NE Goodview Circle, Suite C, Lee's Summit, Missouri, 64064, U.S.A

While they have made every effort to verify the information here, neither the author nor the publisher assumes any responsibility for errors in, omissions from or different interpretation of the subject matter. This information may be subject to varying laws and practices in different areas, states and countries. The reader assumes all responsibility for use of the information.

The author and publisher shall in no event be held liable to any party for any damages arising directly or indirectly from any use of this material. Every effort has been made to accurately represent this product and its potential and there is no guarantee that you will earn any money using these techniques.

ISBN-13: 978-1-7345596-0-6

Table of Contents

Dedication

This book is dedicated to the physicians who are talented and fabulous with so much to share but have not stepped into their highest potential because of fear or because of feeling bound, tied up, restricted.

Here's to you becoming a positive, powerful and impactful "Physician Unleashed."

Epigraph

"You can have anything you want if you are willing to give up the belief that you can't have it."

Dr. Robert Anthony

"Our deepest fear is not that we are inadequate. Our deepest fear is that we are powerful beyond measure. It is our light, not our darkness, that most frightens us. We ask ourselves, 'Who am I to be brilliant, gorgeous, talented, fabulous?' Actually, who are you not to be?"

Marianne Williamson

Personal Dedications

"To the three loves of my life, my husband, Carl and my sons, Myles and Dawson. I am grateful to have all of you in my life. You have watched me work late, travel and participate in meetings at all hours. Thank you for allowing me the space to pursue my dreams and for loving me for me.

To my mom and dad, I am where I am today because of the values you have poured into me. To my baby sister, Shawna, you are beautiful on both the inside and outside. Thank you for loving me unconditionally.

Malaika, you take dreams and make them a reality. You are truly Unlimited!"

Love you all, Tamika.

"To my husband Thaddius, in you I have the sweetest love, the deepest devotion and the strongest support – all beyond what I could have ever imagined. I love you dearly and thank God daily for you.

To my daughter, Khalia and my son, Mekhi, mama loves you and my greatest desire is for you to walk through life boldly, without fear and fully aware of all the wonder and talent that has been placed inside you.

To my mom, dad and wider family, thank you all for always being my cheerleaders. I always felt bold enough to pursue my biggest dreams because you all told me I was special and made me believe I could do anything.

Tamika, in you there is a special light and people are naturally drawn to your brilliance. I am privileged to call you friend. Let's change the world! Thanks for challenging me to dream bigger!"

With love, Malaika

Free Bonus for Readers Only

Are You Ready to Take the Next Step and Become a Profitable Abundant Physician Unleashed?

Because you invested in this book, you qualify for a chance to get a 30-Minute Freedom Formula Discovery Call. The call is designed to give you practical (and easy) ways to grow your practice, have a bigger impact, and take more time off.

On the call, we'll review your current practice (or your plans to start one) and will show you some of the areas where you can instantly create massive growth. We'll also diagnose potential gaps that are preventing you from having the practice of your dreams.

By the time we are done, you will be 100% clear on the next steps you need to take to better your lifestyle, make a bigger impact and get paid what you're worth!

To apply, visit the link below:

www.PhysicianFreedomFormula.com/discovery

Preface

As you're reading this book, we'll assume that you like the idea of being a Physician Unleashed.

In other words, you want to break free from problems such as:

- Insurance restrictions getting in the way of making the best choices for your patients
- The constant feeling that someone is looking over your shoulder
- The fear that at any moment some administrator may give you the ax because you didn't meet their productivity standards
- Working extra hours to see more patients just to make ends meet

Of course, no one thought being a physician was easy. We knew there would be many years of training and we might have to work long and unpredictable hours. But the harsh reality is there is much more to it than that.

Physicians are now having their autonomy ripped from them.

They are being treated like hourly employees and their job security is uncertain.

You have surely heard the stories of physicians employed by large corporations being called into a meeting and informed that they had less than four weeks to find a new job or take a huge pay cut.

Not only that, but the job satisfaction we once looked forward to is often no longer there and the financial pressures can be significant.

When you take all these factors into account, it can be very easy to go along with the idea that the world is changing and that perhaps we have to accept that our career as physicians has turned out different from what we expected.

We're here to tell you that you don't have to fall into the trap of thinking that way.

The reason we wrote this book is to show you that you can make a different choice.

> *The job satisfaction we once looked forward to is often no longer there and the financial pressures can be significant.*

A Better Way

Fortunately, we found there is a better way to serve your patients and build your career. The secret is to build a successful independent practice. This allows you to set yourself free of these problems we've mentioned.

Imagine how different your life would be if you could unleash the time and freedom to enjoy these benefits:

- Spend the time that you need with patients to help them have a better life
- Finish the notes, have all the tests ordered and still be home at the time you want
- Get paid fees that reflect your experience and the changes you bring to people's lives
- Stop worrying about what you need to do to CYA – *Cover Your Ass*
- Forget about having to justify repeatedly why you need the tests for your patients

You'll now have a spring in your step and a genuine smile on your face as you enter your practice doors and you'll be ready to give patients the time and help they need while getting paid accordingly.

While you still have to meet your obligations, you'll escape from the frustration of hesitating to do certain procedures and tests because the reimbursement is so low.

Your judgement is no longer clouded, and your mindset is now, "Let's get it done."

Your family knows that your days are full and you are focused at work, but when you get home, it's all about them and creating quality, fun, unforgettable memories.

It's the formula we used to break free from the stresses of our previous lives.

The kids occasionally say, "I think I want to be a doctor like you.

You own your business, you help people feel better, you make good money and you actually have time for fun with us all the time."

Indeed, you must be doing things right for your kids to want to follow in your footsteps!

Is it a Dream?

We get it. There is some hesitation in your mind as you read this.

This is a dream.

Right?

It doesn't have to be.

What if there was a formula you could follow to make that happen?

The good news is there is such a formula.

It's called the Physician Freedom Formula.

This is the formula we used to break free from the stresses of our previous lives and build successful independent practices where we can help our patients and enjoy the lifestyle we want.

That's what this book is about, so we invite you to follow along with us and become a Physician Unleashed.

Tamika Henry, MD, MBA
Malaika Woods, MD, MPH

SPECIAL BONUS OFFER:
FREEDOM FORMULA DISCOVERY CALL

Because you invested in this book, you qualify for a chance to get a 30-Minute Freedom Formula Discovery Call. The call is designed to give you practical (and easy) ways to grow your practice, have a bigger impact, and take more time off.

On the call, we'll review your current practice (or your plans to start one) and will show you some of the areas where you can instantly create massive growth. We'll also diagnose potential gaps that are preventing you from having the practice of your dreams.

By the time we are done, you will be 100% clear on the next steps you need to take to better your lifestyle, make a bigger impact and get paid what you're worth!

To apply, visit the link below:

www.PhysicianFreedomFormula.com/discovery

Part One: Breaking Free

Chapter 1: Straining at the Leash: Five Reasons Why More and More Physicians are Yearning to Break Free

If you're anything like us, you set out to study medicine believing strongly in the difference you could make in other people's lives.

You also felt you were entering a career that would be highly rewarding in many different senses of the word.

Of course, the world has changed in many ways over recent years, and medicine cannot be immune to that.

But there are many factors that are causing physicians to wonder if they made the right choice or if there is not a better way.

Here are five of the key reasons we find that so many physicians are trying to find a better way forward.

1. Physicians are Becoming Dispensable

In May 2017, Modern Healthcare reported that for the first time ever less than half of physicians were independent.

This was based on an American Medical Association study showing that in 2016 only 47.1% of physicians had ownership stakes in a medical practice.

The same Modern Healthcare article quoted Joel French, CEO of SCI Solutions, a company that offers web-based solutions to connect patients, referring physicians and hospitals, saying, "Physician compensation is one of the fastest-growing expenses in health systems."

It has become as high as 10% of total expenses for some systems. "The burden is not sustainable," French said.

You don't have to wonder what he means by "the burden is not sustainable."

It's likely there will be a deliberate and widespread reduction in the number of physicians in the workforce.

Physicians are being replaced by nurse practitioners, physician assistants and even medical students in some rural areas.

There are experiments going on now to see how much technology can replace services rendered by physicians.

You definitely want to be thinking about these issues, but perhaps you should be doing more than thinking. Should you be taking it a step further and doing something about it?

Are you going to sit idly by and wait for these changes to happen to you?

Alternatively, are you going to sit idly by and wait for these changes to happen to you?

Are you prepared for that Friday morning meeting when you are told that your group is being replaced and you can either stay with a 30% pay cut or get in the unemployment line?

2. Insurance Companies Decide What Matters

Insurance is a great concept. It's a means to help individuals prepare for an unexpected, large cost by paying in small payments over time.

With your car insurance, life insurance, homeowner's insurance, if there was a major problem in any of these areas, your insurance would kick in.

However, with health insurance, somewhere we have gone wrong.

The initiation of managed care is when insurance began to be a barrier to healthcare versus a benefit.

Insurance began to be a barrier to healthcare versus a benefit.

In only a few decades, doctors no longer had the right to make the decisions for their patients. Instead, the insurance company decided what tests should or could be ordered.

Now doctors and their staff have to spend endless hours waiting on hold just to talk with some representative who tells them their patient cannot get the test they so desperately need.

Then what? More paperwork, more time on the phone, more fighting with the system just to do what is right.

This is exhausting. For all involved.

Now we have a new paradigm: PATIENTS FOR DOLLARS.

The old paradigm was first do no harm, which means do the right thing for the patient.

In this new paradigm of medicine, evaluations are based on ability to increase revenue.

Doctors have lost control. A doctor without autonomy is not a good system, and it's not how things should be or were intended.

Under the new system of insurance control, there is more oversight and risk of litigation or accusation of insurance fraud that can lead to jail time.

3. Job Satisfaction is Dropping

For many of us, our journey in medicine typically begins with a simple wish to help people, and part of the reward comes from making a difference in people's lives.

We committed to rigorous training to be able to give our best to those suffering from health issues. But there was also a belief that it would all pay off in the end.

For many, that end was when you put up your sign and said, "New doc here, ready to help those in need."

But the truth is much has changed since we started with the dream of building a career in medicine.

Talk to any long-established doctor, who was practicing in the 1980s, for example, and you will hear the stories about the "good old days."

At that time, most doctors were able to make a good living while helping many people. Patients were more trusting and willing to follow your guidance.

In those days, the doc had a smile on his or her face from seeing the improvement in their patients, and the patients really appreciated the doctor's care and concern. It was a win-win.

Believe it or not, there really was a time when:

- Physicians could spend the time needed with their patients.
- There was less restriction on what a physician could order to help diagnose and treat their patients.
- The patients were able to sit down and have a discussion with

their primary care doctor and/or specialist and take big strides to get their health concerns addressed.

- Doctors had enough time to counsel patients on the steps they needed to take to get better. Patients felt the doctor cared and were more willing to follow their guidance.

In those days medical care was based on what was right for the patient and was not determined by the insurance industry, co-pays, HEDIS (Health Care Effectiveness Data and Information Set) and patient satisfaction surveys.

In short, physicians actually practiced medicine and were well compensated for their time and expertise.

But, oh my, how times have changed.

The growth of insurance-based care has truly taken off and created this push for doctors to see more people in a shorter period of time in order to make a decent salary.

On one level, we now have very little time to help people get better and no funding for preventive medicine. So, we are less able to help our patients truly improve the quality of their lives.

On another level, it's sad but perhaps not surprising that levels of job dissatisfaction and physician suicide rates are at an all-time high. The truth is that being a doctor has become something of a thankless job.

To spend four years in medical school and three to five or more years in residency and then work your ASSets off for what amounts to an hourly rate just above minimum wage seems like a cruel joke.

According to a May 2017 article in *Scientific American*, there is even a club called the Drop Out Club where physicians counsel one another on leaving the field.

To make matters worse, someone who paid a $20 co-pay can ruin your reputation or put you on the "bad doc" list with the insurance company with one bad review.

Now the insurance companies are determining your pay based on how well the patients like you and how many tests you did NOT order.

They don't seem to value all the things you have done, such as all the diagnosis and treatment plans you provided for the other satisfied and non-complaining people who have come through the door.

The majority of satisfied patients who did not take the time to write a positive review are unheard and overlooked.

They don't give you credit for all the times you go above and beyond to ensure the patients get the best care.

There is a lot of time you spend outside of patient contact hours that goes unacknowledged and unappreciated.

You don't get recognition for all those extra hours you spend calling and discussing the case with specialists, reviewing the medications with the pharmacist and ensuring that the patient understands what is actually going on with their bodies.

On top of that, you spend even more time reviewing articles in journal clubs or independently searching PubMed and UpToDate, calling colleagues, and checking Epocrates for drug interactions.

There is a lot of time you spend outside of patient contact hours that goes unacknowledged and unappreciated. How about when you are still in the office after hours charting, while your spouse and kids are texting, calling and asking, "Are you coming home soon?"

Too many of us are missing out on kids' practices, games, spelling bees, and the annual Muffins with Moms and Doughnuts with Dads.

At home, your spouse and you are like ships passing in the night. There is less and less time to talk. When you are home, you are present physically but somewhere else mentally.

Oftentimes, you as the provider are at home reflecting on your practice and what the best next steps are to ensure you meet the demands of the insurance company, address the patient frustrations, and remain hopeful that the reimbursement for services rendered check is on time and a little bigger than the last.

Yet still everyone on the outside looking in thinks we're rich and we have it made because we are doctors. They just don't understand.

When we look at the tired and frustrated faces of our colleagues, we know that so many of them have lost hope and given up.

So many physicians have settled for the employee role and are just working to receive the next paycheck.

This is a sad state of affairs. It's not good for physicians and it's not good for patients. Yes, it is true. Not all providers want to have their own practice and staff and control their own office.

Those of us who are owners of an independent practice have stepped up to the plate, believed in ourselves, and trusted that our practice provides excellent service and patient care. It's time to reclaim the income, impact and lifestyle we so desperately want.

4. The Financial Pressures are Great

To the outside world, it often looks as if we have a relatively easy time financially in the medical profession.

First of all, because patients are paying high insurance premiums, they probably feel there should be plenty of money available.

Second, as we mentioned, most people think doctors are very well paid, even rich.

But the reality is that we live under a great deal of financial pressure both personally and professionally.

On a personal level, a large number of doctors have high loans as a result of going after an advanced degree.

It's not surprising that they say M.D. stands for Major Debt or that D.O. equates to Debt Overboard.

The point is that the expense of training is not typically reflected on the provider's income.

Added to that, as we also discussed earlier, jobs are becoming less and less secure and earning good pay this month doesn't necessarily mean you'll do the same next month.

On a professional level, physicians are being pushed to see more patients every day in order to make financial ends meet.

It's like a restaurant trying to get people to eat faster so they can get new people to the table sooner.

This churn approach of seeing more patients has started to take its overall impact on providers.

There is a sense of bitterness that raises its ugly head as more and more physicians are being told what they can and can't do by those who dominate the insurance world.

Practitioners are feeling the brunt financially of the low rate of reimbursement for services rendered.

There is now a debate of "Should I do this versus that?" based on the craziness that the insurance company may not cover the service and the provider may have to fight for some type of reimbursement.

Slowly the provider gets upset thinking, "We used to make $150 for this service and now we make $30 for this service on a good day."

The bottom line, take-home pay for most medical practices is only about 30%. That means high overhead and little leftover to take home.

Then we see how the patient is caught in the middle of the madness because they are under the false pretense that their insurance covers their healthcare.

5. The Future Looks Even Worse

So, we're painting a picture that circumstances for physicians aren't quite what they were in the "good old days."

The question is whether this is just a temporary blip, or are we seeing a trend that will continue?

It's always tough to predict the future accurately, but many people believe that three levels of healthcare will develop in the future:

- Base tier of government and state-funded plans
- Commercial insurance plans
- Top tier offering a more personalized approach

Let's break these down.

Base Tier
The base tier will be government and state-funded plans. These entitlement programs have already come under great scrutiny.

The funding of these programs is a great expense to our nation and they are constantly on the proverbial chopping block.

We have all heard the discussion for years about whether or not Medicare and Social Security will be available to us when it is time to retire.

Commercial Insurance
The second tier will be commercial insurance plans. In the last few years, we have witnessed the cost of healthcare plans skyrocket.

At the same time, deductibles have also gone through the roof and it is utterly frustrating for both patients and healthcare providers.

In essence, with such high deductibles, patients are unknowingly paying for most of their healthcare out of pocket.

Patients have the false sense of security that they have insurance but don't see the limitations of what it actually covers – high deductibles, high co-pays and high cost for prescription medications.

This becomes an issue because now you, the physician, have to wait for your reimbursement from the patient versus the insurance company.

> *Patients have the false sense of security that they have insurance but don't see the limitations of what it actually covers.*

Because the patient is now responsible for the high deductible, the likelihood of actually receiving payment is lower.

If you have run your own practice or are familiar with the numbers relating to unpaid medical bills, you'll know that getting your payment after the service has been rendered from a patient who may already be strapped for cash is a hefty feat.

This is especially true considering that most families live paycheck to paycheck, and one of the leading causes of bankruptcy and financial strain is healthcare bills.

An insurance-based medical practice generally has to write off 35-40% of medical insurance claims because the insurance company will demand their discount and some patients are not able to pay their balance due.

The entire system seems to be teetering on the edge of a cliff. All the while, both patients and physicians are struggling in this equation, but the insurance companies are making more.

Top Tier

The top tier of healthcare will be for those who are looking for a more personalized approach.

They have more disposable income and they are seeking physicians who have the time and expertise to treat them comprehensively and also offer a top tier experience.

This is the group of patients who are interested and willing to invest in their health and want the best.

One of the decisions you have to make personally as a physician is in which of these tiers you want to build your career.

In this book, we'll focus on the opportunities in the top tier as we believe that's where you have the best potential to build an independent practice and live the lifestyle you want.

We want to be clear that we believe all people should receive healthcare in some form. It is also noble work to treat the underserved. We have both done so at various times in our careers and we continue to give back.

However, this book is speaking to those who have or are planning to start an independent practice.

There Has to be a Better Way

As we said at the beginning of this section, most of us probably go into medicine because we wanted to do well. But the current state of healthcare makes that so hard.

You took an oath to first do no harm, but if you're completely honest with yourself, some days you're not sure if you're even holding up that simple standard.

Your time is so limited and the administration is breathing down your back about being more productive (meaning, see more patients!).

The reality is there is little time to even think about the patient outside the seven minutes you have in the room or the other 30+ minutes it may take you to do the charting and send the prescriptions.

Not to mention the other necessary hoops you must jump through in order to make everybody happy and for you to continue to get paid so you can put food on your family's table.

Because of all the new barriers of low reimbursements, more paperwork, and less revenue per hour, doctors have less time for patient interaction.

One study published in 2018 in the Journal of General Internal Medicine reported that doctors interrupt their patient, on average, after just 11 seconds! Some physicians may just call this statistic being efficient.

The truth is, one of our greatest assets as physicians is to listen to the patient's story, her history and symptoms.

Those items alone will often shed so much light into what is going on with the patient and can be as powerful or more powerful than expensive diagnostic tests.

This simple art of active listening has a major impact on your patient's health journey.

When the doctor is overly concerned with keeping up with insurance and other governing bodies' mandates, he or she has less time to be concerned about the patient's condition.

Now, with only seven minutes per patient, it is much easier to write a prescription for whatever the condition is versus spending time to counsel the patient on lifestyle changes that have been shown in research to be just as effective as medication in some instances.

As a result, patients are getting sicker while doctors are more disillusioned and burned out.

Take a moment and imagine with us. What if?

- You could take the best steps to provide what is necessary for your patients.
- Your administration is focused on high quality interactions and good outcomes instead of emphasizing high volume.
- You get to focus on helping your patients live their healthiest, best lives instead of being on the defensive and constantly worrying about getting sued.

This scenario doesn't have to be a fantasy. Having a rewarding practice is possible.

In the next few chapters, we will share with you how we did it and how you can do it, too.

Making the Change

It's important to note, if you want to build an independent practice where you are not dependent on insurance, you cannot spend the bulk of your efforts competing for the lowest prices.

That means, when we look at the three tiers we mentioned earlier, it's most likely that you will have to focus on the top tier.

You will need to create an experience that demands a higher price point.

For some of us, this may cause a bit of dissonance or tension because we got into medicine to help people.

Yet now we are talking about focusing your effort on helping those who are willing and able to help themselves.

We can say that over time, there is a solution to meeting both of these desires.

However, you must start by establishing a process that grows and sustains your practice. It is important to make sure your business is sustainable.

As the saying goes, put the oxygen mask on yourself first before placing it on others. Though you are here to help people, you are still running a business. Unfortunately, so many physicians forget to manage their business and end up not able to help anyone, including themselves.

Then, as you build your business, you can re-evaluate your time and see where you can go back and help the patients who are not in this tier.

The wealth author, Grant Cardone, says it really is your duty to do the absolute best you can financially so that you can reach back and help others.

As we will explain, you can create patient experience with excellent outcomes in such a way that your patients will be more than happy to pay premium prices for your services. And they will thank you for it!!

Breaking Free

To get started, it may be necessary for you to take a leap and step outside your normal box.

That means you may be required to step outside your comfort zone.

If you know that you have been called for more than just being an employee and if you are ready to make a bigger impact in the lives of patients, we invite you to break free of the leash.

From what we've just covered, it's not surprising that so many physicians are straining at the leash.

So, what's stopping more of us from breaking free and how can we overcome that? We'll look at that in the next chapter.

Chapter 2: Removing the Roadblocks: How to Destroy the 9 Blocks that Could Stop You from Breaking Free

If you want to help your patients in the best way possible, while still enjoying a great lifestyle, it's becoming clear that you need to break free from the restraints holding you back.

For many physicians, that means taking the steps to establish an independent practice free from insurance.

However, it's clear that taking that step is much easier said than done.

There are often mental and practical roadblocks that influence the way we think and work that stop us from fully unleashing our potential.

We've found that these roadblocks tend to fall into one of the following categories:

- Mindset Roadblocks
- Management Roadblocks
- Marketing Roadblocks

Often it takes some effort to overcome these roadblocks, but there is no doubt that not only is it possible, it can also be easier than you realize when you follow the right steps.

Later, we'll talk about the steps you need to take.

But first, let's talk about these roadblocks that get in the way and how they can be overcome.

In the next chapter, we'll go through how we faced some of these issues ourselves when we decided to break free from the old constraints.

Overcoming Mindset Roadblocks

The first category covers the mindset roadblocks, and here are some of the issues that may surface.

1. Face Your Fears and Take Action

One of the biggest issues facing physicians considering breaking free is the existence of fear, which can be represented in a variety of ways, including:

- Fear of failure
- Fear of not having enough money
- Fear of success
- Fear of "getting out there"
- Fear of what others think - patients, family, peers
- Fear of not knowing what to do
- Fear of "my situation is different" or "this won't work for me"

As the motivational speaker, Zig Ziglar, said, "There are two ways of looking at fear."

In one way, it stands for Forget Everything And Run. In this case, we allow fear to hold us back from doing what we know we need to do.

However, another way of looking at it is Face Everything And Rise. We now use our fears to drive and motivate us to take action.

As Zig said, "The choice of which way to view it is yours."

We've faced many of these fears just like others, and we've learned that success only comes when you admit these fears and take action to address them.

It is not surprising that physicians are fearful of the prospect of starting an independent practice, especially since there is nothing in our medical training that prepares us for many of the challenges we must face.

When you are used to getting a paycheck every two to four weeks, life in an independent practice can seem very different.

As physicians, we're comfortable with, okay, do A, then B, then C, followed by D. That's the way that we're used to being trained, but when you venture out to start your own business, there is no clear path.

The problem is that many of us have a fact-finding, researcher-type mentality.

In other words, we need to know the data, the worst-case and best-case scenarios. We want the confidence and backing of randomized clinical trials before we make one move.

This mentality may be fine for some areas of medical practice, but as business owners, too many physicians become crippled with analysis paralysis.

> *As business owners, too many physicians become crippled with analysis paralysis.*

This type of physician likes to think and think and think... and they take entirely too long to act — if they act at all.

Contrary to the popular children's tale of the turtle and the rabbit, the turtle will NOT win this race.

Dr. Woods found this turtle mentality was a problem in the large OB/GYN group she belonged to in the past.

There were many times they needed to make a decision but got stuck because someone needed more data, needed to think about it more and talk it over.

The issue would be tabled, but as the weeks wore on, other seemingly pressing issues came up.

As a result, the important decisions they needed to make were never made, and the business suffered.

As a junior partner in that independent physician-owned practice, Dr. Woods grew frustrated by the inability to make decisions and left the practice. A few short years later, that group is no longer in business.

To be successful in your practice, it's vital not to get stuck in analysis paralysis.

We have to recognize that this is a form of fear that prevents many people from taking action.

We must find ways to recognize the fears we face and then move forward to address them.

As you recognize your fears, you also need to be prepared for some ups and downs. We'll talk later about what we call the independent practice roller coaster. This is an expected part of the process in the world of entrepreneurs.

Sometimes we can enjoy success in the beginning, and then something happens like a dramatic drop in revenue, which can cause us to think about retreating. It's crucial to take steps that keep us moving forward.

The Physician Freedom Formula, which we outline in this book, will help you navigate the process and keep you moving forward.

2. Have the Humility to Learn from the Experience of Others

Taking all of the above into account, one thing you have to figure out right away is how to be humble.

Most doctors do not know how to manage a successful medical practice, let alone an independent practice, free from insurance. So, it's important to learn from others who have run successful businesses, not necessarily medical practices.

A perfect example of this point is the mass exodus of physicians moving from owning their own practices to being bought out and managed by big healthcare organizations.

Sometimes it is the easy way out because doctors do not want to be bogged down with all of the paperwork, details and annoyances of running a business.

But in some circumstances, being bought out is the last lifeline for a poorly managed business that is accruing debt and sinking fast.

Though we all like to think that we are the crème de la crème, the best and the brightest, there is a lot to learn about running a successful independent practice.

In our case, we learned quite a bit from chiropractors, both about business and about alternative medicine therapies.

Most medical doctors believe all they need to do is sign up as a provider for the various insurance companies and hang up their sign.

In no time, they expect their schedules to be full with little effort.

However, from day one, most chiropractors have to work that much harder to get a full schedule without the benefit of having patients automatically being assigned to them.

Many physicians wouldn't think they could or should learn from chiropractors, but when you are stepping outside the box, you have to be ready to learn from anyone who is willing and able to teach you and who has successfully done what you are trying to do.

The reality is that some of our best business teachers and mentors were chiropractors.

Dr. Henry says all the time that we should not have to reinvent the wheel. Learn from other successful people. This goes back to the basics of medicine: See one, do one, teach one.

This also goes back to humility. In the early stages, we were reluctant to invest in others telling us how or what to do. Surely, we were smart and could figure it out on our own. We didn't feel like we needed a lot of guidance – just a little.

Dr. Woods says she was a typical physician cowgirl. A cowgirl is one who just goes for it with no time for too much deep thought and over analysis about things.

She saw herself as more of a do-it-yourself-er who didn't need any help with this.

The way she saw it, as an OB/GYN, you kind of have to be a cowgirl. And she mistakenly thought she could apply those same principles to running an independent practice.

There are some aspects that lend themselves well to being a cowgirl. You try not to overthink things but focus on taking action.

Many times, you suffer unnecessary bumps and bruises because you didn't follow the path that had already been prepared by someone else.

However, there are many times when being a cowgirl can cause you to suffer unnecessary bumps and bruises because you didn't follow the path that had already been prepared by someone else.

On the other hand, Dr. Henry is a researcher. She is trying to thoroughly get an understanding, which, of course, is not a bad thing.

But the issue is, she would continue to look things up, study the methods of other successful providers and not take action.

It was as if she was searching to avoid not taking a step forward. The old analysis paralysis problem.

We both needed to deal with our own roadblocks. Dr. Woods, doing too much, too fast without concern for possible consequences. Dr.

Henry being at times too cautious. The blend of both is more ideal for forward moving physicians. This leads to intentional forward action.

When you think about it, learning to be a physician is about following in the footsteps of those who successfully charted the path before you.

As physicians complete their training and get more independent, this concept of learning from others gets lost, in some cases, because now we can practice independently and have more confidence.

Once you are comfortable and confident in your specialty area, you are at the top of the mountain. It is easy to forget how you got there or how many shoulders you had to stand on to reach the top.

In the same way, when we decided to take a different approach to medicine, we needed to find others who had done it successfully before us.

3. Get the Right People Around You

One of the keys to your success is ensuring that you have people around you who are helping you to move forward.

It's too easy to come under the bad influence for example of:

- Friends and family who say it's too much risk
- Peers who try to tell you it's too difficult or who try to hold you back with their disapproval
- Bad staff who won't go out of their way to serve patients

Equally, a big problem is that many of us try to do too much ourselves, perhaps because we hate the idea of employing people or we want to save money.

As a first step, it's vital to ensure that you only allow yourself to be influenced by people who will support and encourage you.

Of course, we're not saying you should only listen to people who tell you what you want to hear. Candid advice from people with the right experience and knowledge is important. But what can be even more important is to filter what you hear on a daily basis from the people closest to you.

Often friends and family members have no experience of what is involved in building a business, yet they will still make unsupportive comments about what you are doing.

You may find you need to limit interaction with some people in your circle if they are not being supportive.

While that's not always possible, especially with family members, you can choose what information you share about your business, and you can certainly make choices about what you pay attention to.

As we hinted in the previous point, it's important to pay attention to people who have something valuable to add based on their own knowledge and experience.

So, you should actively seek people who have charted the path you want to take. They can advise you on the best steps and help you avoid the pitfalls.

Ways to do that include:

- Hiring a coach, mentor, advisor
- Attending appropriate courses and events
- Joining support groups and masterminds
- Making connections on social media

Our personal experience has been great with all of the above. But our best experiences have been with our hired coaches and mentors.

If you think it is odd to hire a coach or mentor, think about this statement someone shared with us: "If your four-year-old playing T-ball gets a coach and the best athletes and celebrities hire coaches, why wouldn't you want a coach to help you achieve more impact, income and freedom in your life?"

Beyond that, we'd actively encourage you to start building your own team around you as soon as possible. You need to make allowance for this in your budgeting, but you don't need to start with full-time employees.

Building your team allows you to focus on where you can add the most value in your business. As you start to grow your business, you need to allocate time and energy for growth opportunities and not the day to day operations that your team members can manage.

Your job as the leader is to set a vision for your team and to recruit people who will help you reach it.

We've learned that it's much more important to recruit people based on their attitude and their commitment to your vision than it is to look for people based on technical skills alone.

> *Your job as the leader is to set a vision for your team and to recruit people who are going to help you reach it.*

If you find you have recruited people who don't share your vision and are not committed to helping you achieve it, our advice is to have them move on as soon as possible.

That may seem harsh, but your first duty is to serve your family and your patients.

Dr. Henry hired a person based on her excitement to get involved in healthcare and wanted to truly help people with diabetes. She later found out this hire was wrong for the position because the person had a rigid approach and was not a team player. It was her way or the highway.

In other words, if things were not done the way she wanted, she threatened to quit. It was difficult for her to take input from any other team member, including Dr. Henry. She only lasted for three months.

Remember, hire slow. Fire quickly.

Dr. Woods had an employee who left for lunch and never came back! That obviously was not a good fit :)

Overcoming Management Roadblocks

The next category covers the management roadblocks, and here are some of the issues these raise.

4. Make Time to Work on the Business

One of the biggest challenges for all independent practice owners is finding enough time to grow the practice while taking care of existing patients.

This is especially true in the early days when you may be working another job at the same time.

Many physicians find they need to work another job in the early days of establishing their independent practice to ensure they have enough cash flow to meet the monthly expenses, pay certain staff and keep the lights on.

The second job is often needed as they cannot pay themselves from the practice regularly after all the bills have been paid.

Taking that into account, one of the common comments we hear is, "I'm just too busy doing what I'm doing to change what I'm doing."

This is such a common roadblock to success. We often deal with this matter with our coaching clients.

After we have taken the time to analyze the business and discover exactly what their one point of focus should be, sometimes they come back and say, "I'm just too busy. I didn't get it done."

This is such a tragedy. They are caught up in the "noise" of staying busy but not being productive.

They are busy doing things that are unrelated to the one thing that would really move the needle in their business.

When you sit down and have them write out what they're doing with their time, so much of it is simply being wasted.

They are doing "busy work" but not actually working in an area that will move them forward.

They have no clarity or focus on the tasks that will accomplish the goals they are trying to achieve in their personal and professional lives.

For example, if the goal is to get more patients, then they need to designate time each day to doing things that will bring new patients in the practice.

Before you can do that, it's important to sit down and really look at how you spend the time that you say you don't have.

> *It's important to sit down and really look at how you spend the time that you say you don't have.*

We all have things going on and we believe we are too busy to do anything new. But if you were to stop and make a true, honest assessment or audit of your time, what would you discover?

Imagine you had a hidden camera following you around for one day. What would we discover?

- Time wasted on social media?
- Constant interruptions?
- Checking emails all throughout the day?

The question really is, what is this time worth to you?

Do you want to continue saying you're too busy and you don't have time?

You need to control your time and not allow your time to control you.

Are you going to decide that it's time to have your own autonomy, control your own destiny and make a good living doing it?

To achieve that, you need to think carefully about how you spend your time.

5. Take Control of the Finances

Many years ago in medical school, we learned from a financial advisor that physicians are typically high-income earners with low net worth.

Because we are high-income earners, it is fairly easy to get a business loan, compared to other professions. And physicians are not immune to making the mistake of borrowing more than perhaps they should.

Dr. Woods made this mistake when she went out on her own in 2012. She left her practice because she was not comfortable with the high-volume practice and being told she needed to see even more patients.

She was able to acquire a loan for her new practice. She rented a 2500 square foot building and did some major renovations. All totaled, she spent about $35,000 on the build-out alone. Plus, she was locked in for a five-year lease.

Most physicians make the mistake of spending too much money on operating costs, which voraciously eats into the profit margin.

She did not know when she signed the lease that she would be completely revamping her practice. At the time, she was just planning to be a full-time OB/GYN.

But things changed and she did not need all of that space by 2015. In September 2015, she stopped delivering babies and stopped taking insurance. But she was tied in. She did eventually move into a smaller, differently configured space with a conference room, which allowed her to host her own patient education workshops.

Dr. Henry made a wise decision to start her practice by renting space in an OB/GYN's office in Glendale, CA. She moved to a virtual office, and later, after growing her practice, she made the decision to move into a full-time executive suite.

The fact is most physicians make the mistake of spending too much money on operating costs (building, staff, inventory), which voraciously eats into the profit margin.

When Dr. Woods was in the group practice, she noticed that she only brought home about 15-20 cents on every dollar earned. It is very sobering and uncomfortable to know that you have generated nearly a million dollars in revenue, but you only bring home around $175,000.

Dr. Henry always used to joke when working with an employer, "If they're able to pay me $200,000, what do you think they're making?"

If there's five of you and each one of you is making anywhere from $150,000 to $250,000, what is that company making?

Dr. Woods' accountant, who has been a long-time trusted advisor, once told her, "The problem with you physicians is that you only look at the bottom line, what you are bringing home. You ought to pay attention to the top of the profit and loss statement, which shows you how much revenue you generated.

Physicians get comfortable making low six-figures while the companies they work for are making millions.

Avoiding the Revenue Roller Coaster

The key to financial stability is to avoid what's called the Revenue Roller Coaster.

We first heard the term Revenue Roller Coaster at a marketing business conference.

You might even be wondering how two medical doctors ended up at a marketing conference. In the early stages, as we both took the journey into running an independent practice, we also took a journey into "alternative" or non-traditional medicine.

This required attendance at many conferences, online courses, and even a few exams.

In particular, we studied and received certification in weight loss, bio-identical hormone replacement therapy and functional medicine (what we like to call root cause medicine).

After about two years of a rapid pace of ingesting all of this new clinical knowledge and with both of us implementing most of these modalities in our practices, Dr. Woods finally said, "This year, we focus on business."

This was especially important for Dr. Woods because though she started a practice from scratch, she had never taken a business course in her life.

But when she said we were going to focus on business, she didn't mean getting an MBA. Dr. Henry already had that, and she could teach the basics of that training.

The key to success is taking control of your finances so they don't control you.

Rather, we wanted to hear from people who were running successful businesses and we wanted to be around other people like us who were growing businesses and had big goals.

So one day, we were in this business conference, and someone mentioned the Revenue Roller Coaster.

Well, the name pretty much tells the story and we could totally relate. We were all ears because we wanted to know what it took to get off the Revenue Roller Coaster.

The Revenue Roller Coaster starts with habits like paying yourself last, putting everyone else first and trying to generate more money by offering more services.

The result of this process is typically falling deeper in debt. Cash flow is not predictable, which leads to emotional highs and lows related to the bank statement.

The highs and lows of cash flow also provided a false sense of how the business was doing overall.

This can lead to overspending in good months.

You begin to focus on the bank statement and not the profit. Spending exactly what you make, not leaving any profit for yourself or money for taxes.

Sometimes we can get overconfident in our own ideas and set unrealistic expectations. For example, we end up purchasing expensive equipment without a set strategy to generate revenue other than the representative promising you that you will make millions. Ask Dr. Woods. She knows ALL about this!

The key to success is taking control of your finances so they don't control you.

6. Find a System to Follow

Most physicians are familiar with the saying, "See one, do one, teach one."

That is a good strategy when you're learning how to do a procedure.

However, this does not translate well into running a business. Or does it?

Most of us learned how to practice medicine by simply following in the footsteps of those who went before us. Yet when it comes to starting a practice, you may be tempted to make the cowboy move of venturing out without a particular strategy.

If you want to run an independent practice, it will require more than just putting up your sign and setting up a Facebook page.

The right strategy needs to be multi-pronged and include a long-term approach that addresses both the immediate cash flow needs as well as a sustainable cash flow model for attainment of future goals.

If you don't have a roadmap, you will fall victim to the Revenue Roller Coaster.

One of our business mentors told us we should get our business down to predictable numbers. In other words, we should know that if we get so many people in a room, a certain percentage should move to the next step we offer, and from there, a certain percentage should move to the next phase.

For example, we may use a speaking engagement as a means to generate new patients. We should know that if we get 20 people in the room, approximately 40% will move to the next step, which is a paid visit and lab review.

Of those who pay for the visit and lab review, approximately 50% should move on to purchase a program, which is a bundle of visits and other services for a specified amount of time – usually three to six months.

> *The only way to have a predictable business is to have systems in place.*

The only way to have a predictable business is to have systems in place. There is a basic method that any physician can adopt and apply to their practice.

We call it the Physician Freedom Formula. We'll explain that more later in the book.

These concepts are rather simple and basic for business and marketing. They are not hard to understand.

However, as the saying goes, if running a successful business was easy, everybody would do it. It is having the will, discipline and motivation to carry out the easy concepts that is the hard part.

That's why a system is important.

We have found with our physician clients, whom we coach through this process and help with the implementation side, this system is easily implemented and reproducible.

As we mentioned before, we learned from great mentors. At some point, we had to step out on faith.

We saw that they were successful, and they shared with us how they did it. And we implemented, tweaked, and implemented again.

So that's what we're trying to provide for our clients. Again, we see how the old adage holds true, "See one, do one, teach one."

It used to be, "Have you ever delivered a baby? Well, here you see one, now you can do one, now you can teach one."

Now we want to provide something like that for our physicians so they can feel very comfortable, and we support this by having a step-by-step process for them.

Not only is a system important, but being able to adapt to changes needed in the business is also critical for success. Another thing to consider is to think about how quickly you can change course in a smaller, more agile boat versus an ocean liner. The ocean liner may take more time to shift a few degrees whereas a smaller boat can quickly whip across the water in all types of directions.

> *Being able to adapt to changes needed in the business is critical for success.*

We see this scenario play out in the James Bond and other action movies. The small boat comes alongside the big boat and moves across the water easily, and it eventually has some of its fighters come aboard and take down the larger boat. This same concept is true with business.

Reading the biographies of great business owners is a hobby of ours. We have found many great business owners have the ability to be agile within their business, regardless of the size.

Whether it was Steve Jobs of Apple or Sam Walton of Walmart, they were able to make changes and make them quickly for the betterment of the company and in the best interest of their customers.

As physician business owners, we need to think in the same way. We need to adapt and make changes according to the situation and the economic trends in our business.

Overcoming Marketing Roadblocks

The third category covers the marketing roadblocks, and here are some issues to consider.

7. Treat Patients as Clients

In an insurance-based practice, it is unfortunate but true that it often seems that the patient is more of a nuisance in the equation. Because of the time constraints, doctors are forced to see more patients in shorter amounts of time.

Therefore, the actual visit with the patient can be simply a means to an end. Physicians in an insurance-based practice often only have time to talk with the patient just enough to determine the ICD-10 codes so that they can focus on the next step, which is completing the patient encounter note and the billing portion. Then they must move on as quickly as possible to the next patient.

After you see all the patients in the office, you have phone calls, questions from your nurse and prior authorization requests to contend with.

It has been estimated that for every minute spent face-to-face with a patient, the physician needs double that time for paperwork, electronic medical record charting and other tasks necessary to complete the patient visit.

These are just a few of the many items the physician has to contend with in order to get paid and make the administrators happy.

Dr. Woods has been on the receiving end of this "get them in and out" feeling. As she explains:

> *"Back in 2014, I got really sick after a diagnostic GI procedure. I was in the hospital for about 10 days with a resistant strain of bacteremia.*
>
> *Even though all of my doctors and specialists knew I was a doctor, I could tell that by day four, they were spending less and less time with me, but simply making their quick rounds, so they could write their note and move on.*

They were so much in this mode, none of the specialists were talking to one another.

Thank goodness for Dr. Henry, who advised me, because I wasn't thinking that clearly, to call a meeting with the entire team to develop a game plan. It was like every day they saw my temperature spiking again, but no one was really talking about what to do about it.

They had sort of gone into zombie mode — just going through the motions. Now, I don't discount the care that I received overall. It was potentially life-saving. But I definitely needed my own advocates to help me chart the course of that hospitalization."

The point is when physicians feel like employees and are more concerned about stats, numbers, diagnosis codes, and billing, the focus, which should be the patient, gets distorted.

Unfortunately, patients can suffer.

To be in an independent practice, the focus has to be on the patient.

They are not only your patient, but they are your client. It is our responsibility to help them make well-informed decisions as it relates to their health. When we think about the differences between patients and clients, a couple of things come to mind.

- First of all, the doctor-client relationship is not a dictatorship. It is more of a collaboration.
- Second, when you treat patients as clients, the customer service aspect of what you provide is very important.

Too often we hear the story from our patients that their other doctors mocked them, scoffed at them, and basically talked down to them when they presented their concerns or shared information they had found from Google or Facebook groups.

Doctors in private practice need to understand that these "Dr. Google" patients are often their ideal clients.

These are the true health seekers and they are searching for something different. That something different most likely is you!

Respect them and their efforts, give them comfort in knowing that you have done your research and have received additional training so you are equipped to take them the rest of the way.

These patients can only get so far with doing what was recommended in books, Facebook groups and Google searches. They want you to be their trusted advisor.

The fact is there is a big demand for what you are offering.

Patients don't want to depend on insurance companies and there is growing distrust of the current traditional medicine paradigm.

> *Doctors in private practice need to understand that the "Dr. Google" patients are often their ideal clients.*

With high deductibles, people are already paying for their healthcare out of pocket. Since patients are already paying out of pocket, many of them want other choices besides predetermined healthcare algorithms from insurance companies.

It's time for doctors to think outside of the box. You know why? Because your patients are already doing it. They are stepping outside of the box of traditional medicine and opting not to depend solely on the insurance-based model.

They are searching for other ways to get their health needs met.

Of course, if we're going to treat patients as clients, we need to be able to demonstrate the value of what we do.

8. Develop a Plan to Get New Patients Consistently

Once you have taken the leap to start your own practice, it feels pretty good. You feel like a maverick.

Like Neo in *The Matrix*, you've selected the red pill, and now you can really see the world for what it is.

No longer a slave to those damn insurance companies, no more visits with the administration who show you your "numbers," which is just a session to tell you to work harder, faster, see more. And oh, no raises in sight. But now you are independent and free as you were meant to be.

So, you put your sign out and get yourself listed in the local medical directories and you kick your feet up on your desk and just wait for the patients to roll in. Right? Heck no!

The sad news is that some physicians do not understand this. Marketing is the lifeblood of an independent, cash-based practice.

Too many physicians try to apply the business model they used in their insurance practice to their new independent practice.

When Dr. Woods was a full-time OB/GYN taking insurance, she didn't have to market.

She was part of a group of seven OB/GYNs plus two nurse practitioners and she says, "All we had was a listing in the medical directories, the Yellow Pages and we were designated as the in-network providers with the insurance companies."

As she likes to describe it, they had patients beating down the door! Too many to see, in fact. But life is so much different in an independent practice.

We were recently speaking with a physician who had just started her own practice. She understandably was very excited and proud of the move she had made. She had taken the leap and jumped in.

Dr. Henry asked her what she was doing for marketing, and she said, "Nothing."

There was a little silence on our end, and we thought, "Oh my, she does not understand how this works."

As we developed our businesses, we began to understand that there is a science to marketing and attracting the ideal patient-client.

We understood that we had to be clear on who we wanted to help. And saying we wanted to help everybody was not effective.

There is a saying that if you are talking to everybody, you are talking to nobody.

We learned to get into the heads, feelings and emotions of our clients.

Our goal was to understand their needs and speak directly to those needs with our marketing and messaging.

We understood that we had to be clear on who we wanted to help.

This was a whole new ballgame compared to what we did when following the traditional medicine insurance model.

Our bios and websites usually had tons of information to prove how smart we were, but now we needed to focus on the prospective patient-client and their interests and needs.

It was clear there was a method to this madness, and we needed to get a grasp on it.

The beginning of this process felt very much like we were drinking water from a fire hose. There was so much information to ingest.

Now, as medical doctors, we were used to ingesting, processing and making decisions based on complex information.

But in addition, this was a complete paradigm shift compared to how we were accustomed to medical practices working under the insurance model.

The most important conclusion we came to was that marketing is necessary. It's the lifeblood of the practice.

In Part 2 of this book, we'll talk about this element in much more detail.

9. Accept Your Duty to Sell

A big mistake that many physicians make is thinking that because they are smart and have an MD or DO behind their name that patients should be privileged to have them.

Some doctors think, "Well, I am pretty good at what I do. And a lot better than most in my area."

That may all be true. But we like to call that "entitlement thinking."

The fact is all doctors, but particularly those in independent practices, need to actively recruit and educate potential patients.

But we don't like to think of it as selling.

Many physicians are uncomfortable with the idea of selling. Sales sounds sleazy to some people.

The image comes to mind of a scruffy-looking car salesman with greased back hair and a five o'clock shadow, wearing a poorly fitting suit.

The term sales may also conjure up bad memories if someone tried to sell you something at a high price that had little value.

But the truth is all sales isn't bad. We live in a capitalistic society. Sales is a natural part of our transaction of services and data.

Sales is not a nasty word. It is simply an exchange. Something of value given in return for something of value received.

Some like to give sales a softer term and refer to it as energy exchange. But we think you all can handle the term sales.

We use this word because you also need to get a grip on the idea that you are actually running a business.

And the fact is there are certain things that need to take place in order for a business to survive and thrive.

This is another common mistake that physicians make. They don't think they are running a business. They only think in terms of running a practice.

As a business owner and a clinician, there are many factors to consider.

In general, physicians have taken their eye off the ball of running their business, so many medical practices have failed.

This is such an important point that we'll be coming back to it in more detail in Part 2.

Moving Forward

In the first two chapters, we've spent a lot of time talking about the problems and the roadblocks that get in the way of solving them.

In the rest of the book, we'll be more positive and share some solutions to show you how you can break free.

First, we'd like to share with you our personal stories so that you can see what brought us to where we are today and how we addressed the challenges we've mentioned.

Then we'll share with you the Physician Freedom Formula we've developed that gives you a blueprint to unleash your potential.

Chapter 3: Breaking Free of the Leash: The Stories of How We Got Here

In this chapter, we'd like to share a little of our personal stories and how we got here today.

Then, before we go on to show you how you can do it too, we'll share some of the most vital lessons we've each learned.

Dr. Henry's Story

My path to becoming a medical doctor probably started about the same as yours.

My first thought was, "I can't wait to get through these long, damn dry lectures."

As if the nervous anticipation of hitting the hospital floors wasn't stressful enough, I had the pleasure (NOT) of dealing with some power-trippin', over-the-top residents who thought they were the next best thing since sliced bread.

The attendings called me "Henry" and pimped me about random obscure medical facts. I still remember, "What? Henry, you don't know what this is?"

Wait...I digress. I was having a flashback to rounds.

After graduation and with the start of residency, I started to wonder where I would practice after all this was done.

Would I work at Kaiser, join a hospital-based practice, join a private group or go hang up my own shingle? There were so many options combined with so many uncertainties regarding the next best move.

I guess I did what many of us do. I took a leap of faith and believed it would all work out.

Sold Me a Fairy Tale

In my first job, I went to work in a new practice with no patients. I was told this wasn't a problem because they had a plan for rapid growth. They had painted a picture of easy referrals and a quick build up by working with the OB/GYN practice next door. This new practice was supposed to boom quickly because there was such a need for primary care.

However, I quickly realized this practice was not moving in the direction of getting any new patients. They were light years from filling my schedule. I was sold a fairy tale.

To make matters worse, I had to wait eight weeks to get my first paycheck which was only a fraction of what they owed me!!

My thoughts were, "That's for the birds, never again! Forget being a partner in a private practice. I am going to something more established."

Well, you should never tell yourself, "never again." I took another position with a new start-up practice that allowed for flexibility and a very competitive salary.

It was great to say the least. I was a home-visiting physician taking care of the sickest of the sick. I was the eyes and ears of my colleagues in the office, relaying back to them what was happening with the patients in their homes.

We were creating a true all-encompassing practice taking care of fragile elderly patients.

During my time at this company, I accepted the position of regional medical director traveling and overseeing other doctors and nurses. I was so excited and truly loving life.

But what I didn't know was the financial turmoil that was happening behind the scenes. Funds were being misallocated.

At first, I was reassured that things were being turned around and they were going to run a tighter and leaner team. Yeah, right!

In a matter of weeks, my colleagues and I were no longer employed.

The next thing I knew, this so-called thriving medical practice went hasta la bye-bye, and this happened with hardly any notice.

In a matter of weeks, my colleagues and I were no longer employed. We were called into a meeting, and told the company was no longer open and were thanked for our services.

We left the building with a bad attitude and no more checks.

I was upset, nervous and hurt. I thought to myself, "I will never let this happen to me again."

I was determined to have multiple streams of income and not be caught reliant on one source and be in this position again.

I was married with one son and ready to find a job ASAP!

What now?

Within a week, I was working at a skilled nursing facility for a medical group taking care of patients who had been recently, and often too quickly, discharged from the hospital.

Not My Cup of Tea

This was crazy, too! Because when I was in residency, we had a responsibility for patients in various nursing homes.

Each time I would go see my patients, I thought, "This is just not for me, and I would NEVER work in a nursing home for a living. This is just not my cup of tea."

Like I said, never say never.

I did the exact opposite. I began working for the nursing homes and made it work for me.

There was flexibility and again a very competitive salary, and I had time to actually get to know the patients and their families.

It all sounds great, but it's an area you have to be ready for because it is highly litigious. Patients fall and can fracture their hips, and you can get named in lawsuits because you are listed as a provider.

All I would think was, "I wasn't even at the nursing home at 3:30 a.m."

At least I can say I have never been sued and my name has been dropped from any and all cases in the nursing homes.

Something Missing

As I stayed there, I began to realize something was missing in my medical career.

I practiced medicine and for the most part had a great time with my patients, but I often thought, "If I am making six-figures, what is the owner making?"

Like many other physicians, my employer promised me the opportunity to earn a generous bonus. However, I soon realized the ugly truth about these bonuses.

As you may have experienced, these bonuses never come to fruition.

Either the given bonus structure is set where it's unachievable, or you hit the metrics and are told the company is in the red and is not giving bonuses. This really happened to me!

I started to ask myself questions. Why are the metrics unachievable?

Why are we not compensated? If the whole company is not doing well, how did they just buy another building and some other medical groups?

As Arsenio Hall would say, "Things that make you say, 'Hmmmmm?'"

As a physician working in hospital/nursing homes, I was aware there are certain quality of care metrics that had to be met, and I always did my best to make my employer/supervisor look good. This means I dealt with the nonsense.

I dealt with the day-to-day operations and was always mindful of each patient's length of stay. Despite my efforts to make sure my medical director looked good and the patients were well taken care of, my requested time off was denied.

I often thought, "If I am making six figures, what is the owner making?"

What in the world? My supervisor had the audacity to tell me that I was attending too many medical education conferences. So I asked, "What do you want, a bunch of outdated 'dumb' doctors?"

As a result, I was on a mission to find other ways to be financially compensated that allowed me the same flexibility as working in the nursing homes.

I believed there had to be more than one way besides my current situation.

Then, to add insult to injury, they gave a 1-3% raise and no matching funds for retirement. Once you do the math and take out taxes, that raise equated to approximately $12 more per day.

I thought, "There has to be a better way."

Reclaiming Excitement

I was off looking for a new way to reclaim my vigor and excitement for medicine.

The conferences I attended taught me how to change my approach to patient care and help them from a well-rounded perspective.

I stepped out of the world of medicine and ventured into business conferences and mastermind groups.

I kept saying to myself, "Tamika, think. Medicine is a business and you have an MBA. How do you get the best of both worlds?"

My recurring thoughts were, "How can I practice medicine with a low overhead?"

I wanted to impact the lives of my clients without working 12-14 hours a day, without taking hospital calls and without impacting family vacations.

The more I worked for this medical group, the more I began to realize that I was either going to stay there as a salaried employee or take the leap into private practice.

I had to either believe in myself and my ability to have a successful business, or I was going to continue to have these great intentions and big dreams with no action.

Bold Thinking

I was so bold in my thinking about private practice that I was convinced that taking insurance was not an option. I would not allow my hands to be tied by an insurance algorithm on what I wanted to do for patients as it related to improving their health.

Nor was I willing to be held hostage to low co-pays or waiting by the mailbox for the low reimbursement insurance checks.

I refused to see 15 – 30 patients a day in order to meet overhead expenses just to get a decent paycheck.

Needless to say, I had listened to too many unfortunate stories from my physician colleagues about the woes of insurance companies and I saw the frustration on their faces.

Many of my friends and colleagues in medicine were no longer enjoying practicing medicine and missing out on family events, and they were no longer fully present mentally while talking to patients.

So, I asked myself, "How could I apply the lessons learned from my friends and colleagues in both private practice and employed positions to my ideal independent practice?"

How much longer was I going to be caught up in the in-between zone as a full-time employee while at the same time seeing a few patients of my own each month?

Many of my friends were no longer enjoying practicing medicine.

I was working full-time, and then I had the opportunity to lease a small office in an OB/GYN's practice. I was seeing patients there two half days per week.

I was dipping my toe in the water of private practice. This was a hobby at best because, truth be told, I was not fully vested in a full-time private practice. I liked the idea but had not completely set up shop.

Finding Your BS

I was sitting there in one of my business mastermind groups when the facilitator asked the question, "What is the B.S. reason why you are not doing what you should be doing in your business?"

A microphone was passed around the room for each person to answer the question.

Before it got to me, I sat there with a knot in my stomach. I quickly texted my husband, "I need to quit my job!"

He responded with, "OK! Do it!"

I immediately replied to his text with, "I can't move the needle forward for my own private practice if I am an employee."

Then my heart dropped and my hands grew cold. "What have I just texted?"

Then the mic was passed to me and those same crazy words blurted out of my mouth, "I need to quit my job."

I caught Dr. Woods' eye from across the room as I said it, and I could tell she was surprised to hear me make such a bold declaration.

I would be lying if I didn't tell you I was nervous, nauseous and excited all at the same time.

Where should I have my office? What's the name of my practice? Where are the patients going to come from? Where is the money going to come from?

I love the idea of, "If you build it, they will come." But I believe they need some nudging!

The dream went from my thoughts to paper to action. I was constantly reminded, a dream without action is nothing but a great mental image.

Daydreaming does not pay your bills or feed your family. Momentum and action get you that much closer to the dream in your head and the plan on paper.

I may have started out like a turtle, but let me ask you, what does the fairy tale say about who wins the race? I know we told you earlier that the turtle does not win, but just go with me on this analogy!

Start of Something New

Unlimited Health Institute was born.

- I did not take insurance.
- I did not work on Fridays.
- I would not see more than eight patients per day.

These were all my choices as I set up my ideal practice.

As I dabbled in the independent practice sector, I made $65,000 in the first year. Then I started to really see some changes as I began to embrace my practice.

- At the beginning of my first full year, I hired my first full-time staff member.

- I followed the idea that marketing is the lifeblood of a business, and I went all in with a marketing campaign to bring in new patients.

- I quickly added a second staff member.

- Before I knew it, my days were at capacity. It really was a whirlwind and an exciting time.

I remember my best month of the year was when I had taken one week off in the summer for a family vacation.

Finally, I was seeing the many things I had heard about come to fruition.

- I was making more money without having to work harder.

- I broke the $100,000 in a month barrier while taking time off.

- By the end of the year, I had 10x'd my business. That's $650,000! And the insurance companies didn't get a dime!

It all was possible after I made the decision to fully commit.

I feel that's not too bad for less than 18 months in practice.

Dr Henry's Key Lessons

Let me share with you the top lessons I learned from my experience:

- Stay committed to your dream.

- Keep your thoughts and life positive when you are trying to fulfill your dreams.

- Keep your overhead low.

- Hire slow, fire fast.

- Track your marketing dollars spent.

- Be flexible and willing to adjust quickly.

Dr. Woods' Story

My journey onto the road less traveled began in 2011. At this point I was six years into a very busy OB/GYN group practice, doing what should've been my dream job.

I had wanted to deliver babies since eighth grade, and there I was, a full-time OB/GYN.

But for some reason, I felt unfulfilled. I was seeing 30-35 patients every day and my group was telling me I needed to see more. I was not given the opportunity to really get to know my patients and I felt like I was not practicing good medicine.

This was not what I had signed up for.

In 2011, I was also one year out from having my second child, a healthy, happy baby boy.

One day I stepped on the scale, and it said 236 pounds! I was not happy. I was tired, crashing in the mid-afternoons, barely making it through my hectic workdays.

When I finally got home at night, I didn't have much energy left to really engage with my husband and two beautiful children.

I felt guilty, but yet I was exhausted. My only comforts were the couch and what I could find in the fridge or the pantry.

I was in a vicious cycle that I know so many physicians experience.

To top it off, I felt really ashamed. How could I talk to my patients about getting healthier when I was on the wrong path?

Something had to change.

I was finally sick and tired of where I was. I put my mind to work and started taking courses on weight loss.

I even got board certified in non-surgical weight loss management with the American Board of Obesity Medicine.

In the process, I lost 60 pounds between 2011 and 2013.

I felt empowered and I wanted to share what I had learned with as many patients as possible.

During this process, I left my group and started a solo OB/GYN practice in 2012. In 2013, I added a small, cash-only weight loss clinic. My journey into weight loss then led me into bio-identical hormone replacement therapy (BHRT) certification.

Once I incorporated BHRT, I started seeing great improvement in my clients' health and my cash practice began to grow. But there was still something missing.

One day, Dr. Henry mentioned something about functional medicine, and I said, "What is that? I've never heard of it."

How could I talk to my patients about getting healthier when I was on the wrong path?

She explained that Integrative Functional Medicine is all about discovering the root cause of illness and chronic disease. I quickly realized this was the missing piece for me and my practice.

As I was taking the coursework in Functional Medicine, my cash practice started to overtake my insurance practice. I took the bold leap in September of 2015 to stop delivering babies and to stop taking insurance. I also earned my practitioner certification with the Institute for Functional Medicine.

Now I felt like my toolbox was complete to help patients discover the underlying cause of their conditions and truly unlock their body's AMAZING potential.

I am proud to say that I have run a thriving independent practice with no insurance for the last four years.

It was so exciting to see my revenue jump by an additional $200,000 in just one year after implementing the strategies Dr. Henry and I learned together.

Because I was seeing such amazing results in my own health and my patients' health, I couldn't keep this to myself!

Over the past several years, I have spent hundreds of hours in research and training, not to mention about $100,000 invested in conferences, certifications, coaching and mastermind groups.

Now I feel it is my duty to help unleash other physicians from the daily grind of insurance-based practices with too much work, not enough pay and very little reward.

The Best Strategies

As we continued our process, what first seemed like drinking from a fire hose became a manageable sprinkle. We were able to pull out the pieces and strategies that worked best. We experimented.

Some things worked, and some things didn't. In the end, a system began to develop. Like magic ink, the words and the system began to appear.

Dr. Henry was getting consistent results in California and had her first $100,000 month, and I was getting consistent results in Missouri and had my best year ever in solo practice, even better than when I was taking insurance.

We had our Eureka moment. It's working! It's really working!

Teaming Up

We have developed a passion for helping physicians to become unleashed.

- An unleashed physician is one who is free to help as many people as possible without the restraints of insurance companies.

- An unleashed physician lives an abundant life while at the same time running a successful, fulfilling practice.

To help more physicians become unleashed, we decided to team up and help other doctors with the system we discovered.

That's also our aim with this book.

Dr. Woods' Key Lessons

Let me share with you the top lessons I learned from my experience:

- Never stop believing in yourself.

- Make time to work on the business, not just in the business.

- Fast-track your success by learning from others.

- Remember that failure is an event, not a person.

- Push through the tough times. If you don't give up, you will succeed!

Chapter 4: Making the Big Decision: Taking the Leap

The single biggest block to creating an independent practice is making the decision to take the first step.

Deciding to break free from insurance-based practice is a bit like a game of double-dutch.

If you have ever seen the really great double-dutchers, they make it look really easy.

But if you have ever tried it, you know that it takes skill. When you're new at it, one of the first big challenges is simply getting "in."

Have you ever been there?

Standing off to the side, watching those two ropes swing around and around.

Noticing that every so often, there is an ever so tiny moment where the path is clear and you can jump in.

Then you have to calculate what foot to jump in on and how fast to start jumping once you successfully get in between the ropes.

Taking the leap with a cash practice can be like trying to double-dutch.

The problem with a lot of physicians, and you may have seen this type on the playground back in the day, is that many get paralyzed with just the very first move – jumping in.

We each had our moments of being the paralyzed double-dutch amateur.

Dr. Woods talked about transitioning to cash and giving up OB for about one year before she actually jumped in.

Dr. Henry dabbled with her own practice for two years before that day she described in the business mastermind group, where she said, "I need to quit my job."

And she committed to making that bold move in six months from the day she uttered that declaration.

So, are you ready to take the leap and become a Physician Unleashed?

In the following pages, we share some worksheets to help you decide:

- Are you fed up enough to leap?

- Are you clear what you are leaping to?

When you're ready to join us, we'll see you in Part 2, where we share the roadmap we followed.

SPECIAL BONUS OFFER:
FREEDOM FORMULA DISCOVERY CALL

Because you invested in this book, you qualify for a chance to get a 30-Minute Freedom Formula Discovery Call. The call is designed to give you practical (and easy) ways to grow your practice, have a bigger impact, and take more time off.

On the call, we'll review your current practice (or your plans to start one) and will show you some of the areas where you can instantly create massive growth. We'll also diagnose potential gaps that are preventing you from having the practice of your dreams.

By the time we are done, you will be 100% clear on the next steps you need to take to better your lifestyle, make a bigger impact and get paid what you're worth!

To apply, visit the link below:

www.PhysicianFreedomFormula.com/discovery

Worksheet #1: Are You Fed Up Enough to Leap?

First thing to consider is whether you are really unhappy enough with your current lot in life to take this leap. We're not going to pretend it's easy so you have to be ready to make the commitment.

Read the following statements and rate each between 0 and 10 depending on how strongly you agree, where 10 = Strongly Agree and 0 = Strongly Disagree.

	Score 1 – 10
1. I regularly work longer hours than I would like.	
2. My home life is suffering because of the hours I work.	
3. I am frustrated about having to work such long hours.	
4. I feel that my current job is insecure.	
5. My patients often are not able to get the level of care I would like for them.	
6. I feel some of the people I work with are not always committed to the best patient care.	
7. I feel the hourly rate I am paid is not a fair reflection of my training and value.	
8. I am sick of seeing so many patients in one day and being expected to see and do more.	
9. I don't feel I have enough time to spend with each patient to help them make the changes necessary to get better.	
10. I am sick of being on call.	
TOTAL	

What your score means:

- < 30: Maybe life is not so bad where you are. Are you sure you're ready for the leap? You may not be ready for the leap, but join us in Part 2 to learn what is needed when you're ready.

- 30 – 50: Are you sure you're not just having a bad day or are you really ready? Keep reading. Go to Part 2.

- 51 – 75: You're too close to settle now. Join us in Part 2 and start making your plans!

- 76 – 100: You are ready. Join us now in Part 2 and start looking forward to a better future!

Worksheet #2: Are You Clear What You're Leaping To?

Before you take the leap, let's get clear about what the future should look like.

Stop now and think about it. What dream do you have for you, your family, your lifestyle, and your income? What type of impact do you want to have in life?

Many of us may be thinking about the immediate impact of increasing our bank account and freeing up our time.

Others may simply want to practice good medicine and have a financially sound practice.

There are many different success stories. What matters is what success looks like for you. Take some time now to describe what your reality will look like in the next five years. Think about:

- What type of impact you want to have

- What your practice/office will look like

- How many people you'll employ

- How many hours you'll work

- How many patients you'll have

- How much money you'll earn

- What your lifestyle will look like

- How much time you will take off for family time/vacations

- At what age you want to retire

- Where you will travel to throughout the year

- What your retirement and savings account balances will look like

- What type of relationship you will have with your spouse and kids

- What you will do in your free time

Feel free to write exactly what you want in these areas of your life. This is just for you. There is no judgement on the answers.

Now that you have answered the questions, start to visualize how each of these goals will be manifested in your life. What will it look like? How will it feel?

The next step is to write out your future as if it has happened. This is called future scripting.

Act like you are a reporter, doing a day-in-the-life of YOU five years from now. Write this out based on the answers to the questions above.

Be specific. Describe what your life is like in detail and describe how you feel.

Take 15-20 minutes and do this. You have to dream it to achieve it. A common practice of successful people is their ability to visualize their future before it happens. For more information on this topic, check out the book, *Psycho-Cybernetics* by Dr. Maxwell Maltz.

Part Two: The Freedom Formula

Chapter 5: Introducing the Physician Freedom Formula

In the first part of this book, we've focused on the challenges we face as physicians and talked about some of the steps necessary to break free from them.

In the next section, we're going to focus on the process of breaking free – the steps you need to go through to become the Physician Unleashed.

We personally went through that process with much trial and error, many bumps and bruises along the way, and after about $100,000 each spent in trainings, mastermind groups, workshops and one-on-one coaching.

What we've realized going through that process is that it doesn't have to be as daunting and as complicated as it seems.

The good news is that there is a formula that any physician can follow to break free.

We like to think of it as a nearly foolproof method to build, sustain and thrive in a truly independent practice. We wish we'd known it a few years ago, but we are happy to share our Physician Freedom Formula with you.

The Freedom Formula is simply:

$$A \times V \times S = Freedom$$

The key elements of this are as follows:

A is Authority

Authority is the reputation you have in your community that makes people want to work with you rather than you struggling to fill your schedule.

Authority comes partly from your expertise and knowledge, but it also depends on you taking action to share your message with your target audience (your ideal client).

We'll show you the key elements of establishing authority and the steps you need to take to make sure others know about your expertise.

V is Value

There are two components of value in our Physician Freedom Formula.

The first is that you must believe you are worth what you are asking your patient to invest.

Remember, before you can deliver value to the patient, you first must **_know_** you are worth what you are going to charge. So, we'll talk about dealing with any head trash that may tell you otherwise.

The second part of value revolves around what you deliver to the patient.

We'll talk about how to develop your offer so that people want to invest in it.

Creating an experience that is top-notch and unlike any other doctor's visit your patient has had in the past also creates great value.

It's important to take into account that what you are offering is not a matter of symptoms leading to a prescription for pills. But rather a comprehensive approach with transformational outcomes resulting in a great experience for your clients.

When you deliver value on all these levels, you make it easy for people to pay you fees that reflect what you are worth without having to depend on insurance.

This is the foundation of a strong independent practice.

S is Systems

Systems are the processes you put in place to ensure you have a steady stream of patients and you deliver your services in an effective and profitable way.

We'll work step by step through some of the key systems that will drive your success.

The Formula Story

We came up with the Physician Freedom Formula because it's easy to remember and clearly identifies the important elements.

We are all in favor of finding the easiest way to explain ideas. In medical school, we both always tried to use acronyms and mnemonics that helped us remember the concept more easily.

We felt it was important for our fellow physicians who want to break free and to establish an independent practice to have a formula they can follow that is simple, quick and relatable.

So, let's dig into each of the elements of the formula.

Chapter 6: Authority – Why and How to Get Ideal Patients to Seek You Out

To build a successful independent practice, you must have your ideal patients actively seeking you out as the person who can help them solve their problem.

You certainly don't want to come across as someone who has to aggressively push yourself on people. They should be able to easily discover you as the solution to their problem and seek you out.

The key is being seen as the authority in your field.

You may think that, in other people's minds, physicians automatically have authority. It's partly the white coat, and it's partly the title and qualifications and partly the environment. Those immediately establish the physician as the medical authority in the room.

It's true that patients will often defer to what their physician says. But that comes about when the person is already in front of someone they have decided to trust.

That's where you want to be. People should come to you predisposed to trust you and follow your advice.

Why Authority Matters Now More Than Ever

However, these days, there are many reasons why it's not easy to establish that position up front. For example:

Patients are Losing Confidence in Traditional Insured Medicine

Many patients nowadays hesitate to trust their traditional medical practitioners because they feel their physician's decisions are being dictated by insurance companies and not by what is right for them.

They feel they are going to be told that what they believe they need isn't covered. Patients fear they will fall into an insurance algorithm which predetermines the next test, medication and/or specialist they can see.

Patients feel they are not seen as individuals but rather as insurance codes and are treated like just another number.

Because of this growing distrust and lack of confidence, more patients are turning to alternative therapies.

A November 2016 article in the *New York Times* reports that, according to the National Center for Health Statistics, $30 billion is spent on alternative therapies and supplements each year because patients are looking elsewhere for answers.

People Have Access to the Plethora of Information Online

Patients have access to information now more than ever before, and they are attempting to improve their health with the help of Facebook groups, Instagram, Pinterest, YouTube and Google searches.

People often have their own ideas up front and then look to find all the information that supports what they believe is the right way to go.

Of course, we know some of that information is not always correct and we can joke about patients getting help from Dr. Google.

But it's not necessarily a bad thing to have patients who are well-informed and are asking lots of questions.

Though they may be having some success in their search for information, the truth is they are often still at a loss. They are throwing arrows in the dark trying to make sense of what is going on with their health and their bodies.

They are overwhelmed by information, and they are desperate to find someone they can trust to help them sift through it all and distinguish the good from bad. That someone is *you.*

Because there is so much information available, patients are suffering from information overload. They soon realize what they are finding online is not customized to them specifically.

That's when patients get overwhelmed.

In those instances, when patients present their own research, we may feel challenged or irritated. We may be quick to defend our authority.

But, believe it or not, it is actually very overwhelming for patients who feel they need to do all of their research on their own. They are coming to you with the research because they need your help to sort through it all.

Our job is to facilitate their research, guide them through the vast sea of information and give them guidance.

Information alone is not enough. We believe guided action plus information equals transformation. That's why your authority and expertise are so important.

We see so many people in our practices who come in saying something like, "It's just too much information. I don't know what to do. Do I drink milk? Do I not drink milk? Do I do a ketogenic diet or do I do Paleo?"

Too often, they are thinking, "Well, I might as well not do anything because what I'm doing now is not working. I was following an online health person, and it worked for a little while. But then it stopped."

We always commend people who are being proactive and take steps to move in the direction of improving their quality of life and longevity. They want more guidance and direction from physicians who are confident and ready to lead them to the results they so desire.

Other Sources of Medical Advice are Growing

There's a big boom right now in all sorts of medical advisors, such as health coaches. While they are not supposed to diagnose, often they are doing just that. They are providing treatment plans for patients based on lab results you would think only physicians could order.

In some cases, problems arise that can no longer be addressed by the health coach, and then the patient comes back to you, the physician, for help.

People are reaching and grabbing at so many different things, and they don't have a system or a guide.

We often have patients come in with a bag full of bottles and say, "Here is what I have been doing and here are all the supplements I'm taking."

We Are Needed More Than Ever

It's interesting to see there are many people stepping outside the traditional insurance model, looking for help.

That may be a professional concern to us in some ways. Yet it also shows there are people who have resources and are willing to invest in their health in order to find a solution.

The opportunity to step outside traditional medicine is wide open if physicians will step up.

The truth is many patients are searching for someone in whom they can trust.

Often they just want someone they can trust to take the lead and say, "If you're having this problem, here is my recommendation."

They are looking for those doctors who are qualified, confident and able to make a difference in their lives.

The time is also very ripe for physicians who are sick of their hands being tied by insurance companies. This is a great time to step outside the box and work with patients who are also frustrated.

Why We Hesitate to be the Authority

Despite this underlying demand for expert help, we as physicians often hold back from stepping into our authority.

Why do we do this? There are certain fears that hold us back from stepping into our authority, including:

Personal Reluctance

Many of us hesitate to put ourselves forward as experts as we don't want to come across as arrogant.

Some physicians may feel they are not qualified. You may think, "I can't be the authority figure. I don't have a book. I don't have a TV show. I'm not Dr. Oz."

But the fact is, you are an expert. If you think about it, there is an area of medicine that you can speak on right now without the need for any additional research or the need to read any articles. You talk about it every day with patients.

You have to start believing that it's your duty to share what you know with others and to show them how they can improve their lives.

By hiding your expertise from them, you are doing them a disservice.

In the book, *Winning Through Intimidation*, Robert Ringer talks about the Leapfrog Theory where he says, "Every human being possesses the inalienable right to make a unilateral decision to redirect his career and begin operating on a higher level at any time that he and he alone believes he is ready."

The idea behind the Leapfrog Theory is that you don't waste time making your way step by step up the ladder. You jump immediately to the place that is right for you.

Now, of course, that doesn't mean making claims you can't substantiate and you have to follow the law and professional ethics.

But what it does mean is that when you are holding yourself back, there is someone out there with less expertise than you who is positioning themselves ahead of you in the line to advise your potential patients. They don't hesitate to position themselves as the experts in their field.

You have to imagine that there is somebody out there talking to your potential patients and giving them advice that is not right for them.

It is your duty to make sure that people who need your help know about you.

When Dr. Woods started out, she had to get over the fear of, "Would anybody really listen to me?"

She says, "When I got over the doubt about whether or not I was an authority figure, I found that it was really quite enjoyable to be able to help people simply by shining a light on their health concerns. I'm allowing them to see it from a different perspective. I'm also giving them some validation for having an opinion that's different from the traditional medical approach."

So, once you embrace the idea of, "Yes, I am an authority" and, "Yes, I can help people by owning that position," then it's great and beneficial because you have people come to you and say, "I'm so glad that I was able to hear this."

When we're giving free talks and people sign up for our programs, people often say, "I'm so thankful because now I can get off of Google." They've been doing all the research themselves, and they finally feel they have found someone who can truly help them.

Fear of Peer Group

Sometimes, as professionals, and perhaps especially as medical professionals, we look towards our peer group rather than our potential audience when we ask the question, "Who am I to be an authority?"

In this instance, physicians are not thinking of patients when they ask, "What will my professional colleagues think of me?"

When Dr. Woods decided to start an independent practice, she found herself regularly thinking, "I'm an OB/GYN. I'm venturing out into something different. My colleagues are going to think I'm crazy."

We as physicians often pay too much attention to what our peers think.

We're like, "I don't have the published articles, the hospital acknowledgements or the coveted position of president of the hospital board."

When you think about the relationship with your potential client or patient, you definitely have authority.

To help you own your authority, first of all, it requires some observation.

The fact is, many people desperately need and want natural solutions for their health or some other sort of alternative.

Now you're seeing people who are questioning their traditional doctor because they don't want to take all of the recommended medications. They're saying there's another way. There's an alternative. I don't have to go the traditional route.

The problem is they're out there reaching and grasping for anything. They're talking to the teenager at the general nutrition store trying to get some kind of medical advice.

So, if an actual medical doctor would step up and say, "Hey, I've got a little information on this, and I can help you," people would be so grateful for that.

The first thing is to have the right perspective. People need your help.

Next, it is imperative that you stand up for yourself. You must tell yourself, "I'm not going to worry about what my peers have to say. I'm going to boldly step forward to help people that I know need to be helped."

Most importantly, you have to believe that what you're doing can transform lives.

> *You have to believe that what you're doing can transform lives.*

What you are really trying to do is help patients see you as the authority and make it easy for them to find you.

You are trying to help them make better decisions for their health.

If they see you as the authority and they trust you, there is a better chance they will follow your recommendations.

We believe it's important to spread the message that there is a different way to approach medical issues. There is also plenty of evidence ($30 billion worth!) that people want non-traditional options and will pay for it. Potential patients just have to know we exist.

Lack of a Plan

One of the biggest blocks to stepping into our authority is the fact that we don't know how to present ourselves as an authority.

There are certain processes and tools you can use. We'll cover these next.

The Physician Authority Formula – 5 Keys to Being Seen as the Authority in Your Market

In order for you to become an authority as a Physician Unleashed in your community, you don't have to be as famous as Oprah. You need to look at it in a different way.

There are some keys to authority that you need to bear in mind. Based on these, we can then work out a step by step plan for building authority.

The key elements to authority give us the Physician Authority Formula, which is:

$$Authority = E^5$$

The five elements are:

- **Expertise**: Focusing on a specific area where you can be the expert

- **Empathy**: Understanding the needs and problems of your potential patients

- **Education**: Building trust by providing helpful information to potential patients

- **Evangelism**: Being ready to share your message with your audience

- **Evidence**: Having proof of results achieved by patients through case studies and testimonials

Let's look at each.

Expertise

The foundation of your authority is your expertise. One of the keys to positioning yourself to make the most of your expertise is to recognize you can't be an expert on everything and you normally can't be an expert everywhere.

The fact is you don't necessarily have to be a nationally recognized expert.

It is more achievable to be an expert on a specific topic, and it is often best to do that within a particular geographic area.

Over time, you may find that you start to work with people in a wider area of the country or even beyond. But it's usually better to start by becoming known as an expert in your local community.

When you choose a specific topic, you can concentrate your efforts on knowing as much as possible about that topic. Often you will achieve more by drilling down in your specialized niche.

Let's say you decide your topic is weight loss. It may be better to focus on weight loss for a specific group of people, such as women.

Many physicians are reluctant to be too focused as they feel it means they may miss out on potential patients.

If you can drill down on a specific group, your audience will be more defined and your message will have a greater impact.

For example, that could be helping women with weight loss in a particular age group or with a particular issue, such as recently having had a baby. This is how you define your niche and your area of expertise.

Alternatively, you can focus on specific methods of dealing with weight loss. You can narrow your focus in different ways based on who you work with or exactly what you do.

There may be many practitioners talking about weight loss medicine, but they're not necessarily out there establishing themselves as an authority in their current community nor focusing on specific elements of the community.

Think about it from your own perspective. If you were struggling with postpartum weight gain, would you prefer to get advice from a generalist who claims to know about a wide range of areas, or would you seek help from someone who was an expert in postpartum weight loss?

However, many physicians are reluctant to be too focused as they feel it means they may miss out on potential patients. But the truth is that being more specialized has considerable benefits:

- It is easier and more believable to be an expert in a specific area.

- You can identify and reach your target audience more easily.

- Specialists are more highly valued and can charge more.

Obviously, you need to choose an area – both in terms of geography and specialty – that is big enough to support an independent practice. Many physicians are reluctant to specialize and end up being too broadly based, so they fail to take full advantage of their expertise and authority.

If you want to become a Physician Unleashed, you have to be specific about what you will offer and who you will help.

Empathy

Empathy is the ability to understand and share the feelings of another. With an empathetic relationship, you as the expert can help your patients reach the results they need to achieve.

As an expert, you can come across as knowing better than them and telling them what to do. This may even get results some of the time, but it's not the ideal approach.

Equally, you may have an approach that is too laid back, especially when they are paying you fees, and you won't help them as much as you could.

This has the potential to have a negative outcome because, if you do not hold your client accountable, there is a higher likelihood they will not achieve their health goals and they may walk away thinking your program didn't work for them. When in reality, you didn't hold their feet to the fire to make the changes necessary to achieve their health goal.

Empathy is about getting the balance right in the way you establish your authority.

In a sense, it is about making the patient feel that you are on the journey with them rather than just taking charge, and this will help create a more effective long-term relationship.

The key elements to this are:

- Communication
- Confidence
- Certainty

Communication

A big part of empathy is how we communicate with people. You need to let them know you understand how they feel.

You need to speak to them in a way that is easy to relate to with no doctor jargon. As physicians, many people come into the office preoccupied with what's going on in their bodies and wondering if they are alone, crazy, or broken. We are there to provide reassurance. We need to tell them they are not alone, crazy or broken.

Patients need to feel that your priority is to help them get results.

Often the mere validation of their worries creates an immediate sense of relief and a welcome breath of fresh air. This is how you use empathy to establish trust with a patient/potential client.

Confidence

Next, it's important to give them confidence in the relationship. They need to feel that your priority is to help them get results. It's important not to treat patient appointments as transactional and not to come across as only being in it for the money.

As independent practitioners not held back by the restrictions of insurance, one of the ways we can convey how much we care about them and their health concerns is through the time that we spend with them.

This builds a sense of caring and trust. Ultimately, patients want to work with physicians they know, like and trust!

Certainty

The third element of empathy is certainty. You should start with the assumption that people want to hear your advice.

They also want to know that you have confidence in what you say.

People want to work with the best, especially when it comes to their health. So, be ready to step up to the plate and demonstrate that you are indeed an authority.

Stop undervaluing the importance of what you know and believe that YOU are one of the BEST!

When you act with certainty and give clear instructions, you are helping the patient get results.

This confidence is not cockiness and arrogance, but rather it is consistent with being a leader, an expert and an initiator.

But it's communicated in a way that shows respect and understanding for the patient.

Patients are not looking to work with a physician who walks around timid, uncertain and without confidence.

They are seeking help from the physician who is the authority on the topic and who actually cares to address their concerns.

Patients will not expect you to have ALL the answers, but they should feel that you know your area of expertise well.

Education

An important aspect of being an authority is sharing your expertise with others. One of the most effective ways to do that is through what is called education-based marketing.

In doing this, you share helpful information with people to help them understand more about the problem they are facing.

There is a familiar adage in marketing that people will purchase from someone they know, like and trust. So, it's important that you put in place a system that helps you move prospective patients through a process to know, like and trust you.

Education-based marketing is a great way to achieve this goal.

For example, you might share with a potential patient the root cause of their problem and other areas that need to be investigated.

After you have educated them about the possible causes of their problem, they will be more than eager to hear about how you can help them solve it.

> *It's important that you put in place a system which helps you move prospective patients through a process to know, like and trust you.*

You can provide education-based marketing through a variety of methods that we'll cover in a moment. However, the key is that you start building a relationship with them by sharing information and educating them before they become patients.

Some physicians are reluctant to do this because they feel they should not be giving such knowledge away for free or they feel that giving too much information in this way can be dangerous if people don't understand it fully.

With well-crafted education, you will establish yourself as the authority, and it will be clear to them that you are the person who is ready, willing and able to help them.

If we own up to our authority, we can help many more people. Patients want someone to guide them regarding their health decisions, and they often feel more comfortable if it's actually a doctor who has the willingness, expertise, time and compassion to assist them.

Otherwise, as we've highlighted, your prospective patients are seeking health advice from non-medical people or other online sources without guidance.

None of them have as much training as a medical doctor and people have the most confidence in the information they receive from a physician.

Physicians have the ability to bring together the best of their traditional training combined with natural approaches, and this is highly valuable. Patients will step outside the box and the confines of insurance and gladly pay because they are searching for something greater for their health.

The role of physicians in providing education to help people make the right choices to improve and enhance their quality of life has never been more important. You are highly valuable and you will be sought out.

Education Formula

When we are in front of patients and encouraging them to take action, we follow an additional formula called the E3 Education Formula™ (Trademark: Dr. Woods Wellness).

Here's an example of how we share these key elements with patients:

- **Enlighten.** The first step is to shed light on the problem by asking the right questions and ordering the right tests based on the Integrative Functional Medicine paradigm. Once you become enlightened or, in other words, informed about what exactly is going on in your body, only then can you start to make the necessary changes to correct it. *This is part of the education piece.*

- **Empower.** After the right questions have been answered and the appropriate tests have been done, giving you the tools regarding how to change what is found on the specialized tests is so empowering. Finally, you start to regain control of your health and realize it wasn't all in your head. *This is where you give them validation and respect their opinion.*

- **Energize**. Once you have asked the right questions and determined the answers and the solution, you will not only feel you have more energy physically, you will also be energized mentally and emotionally. With more clarity in every aspect of your life, hope and optimism will be your new normal. After completing the E3 Method, you will learn to age with grace, freedom and fun! *Here we give them hope and get them excited about the possibilities.*

These steps of education-based marketing can be applied to get your prospective client excited about what you can offer and how you can help them. Use this as an example and create your own!

Evangelism

It's not enough just to be an expert in your field. You have to be seen as an authority in the eyes of your prospective patient.

People that you can help should know about you, and it's your duty to reach out to them.

We choose the word "evangelism" deliberately because if you have chosen your area of expertise correctly, you will be really motivated to share with as many people as possible how you can help them.

So, you need to work hard at getting your message across.

To evangelize your message, it is important to have a platform to share your knowledge and expertise.

You don't have to be on national TV to get your message to the masses. There are certain things you can do right now in your local market to let people know how you can help.

There are enough clients who need your services. They just don't know you exist.

You can create your own mini media empire. It does not require millions or even thousands of dollars.

There are free, simple tools you can use, such as:

- Your own website or blog

- Articles in external publications (online and offline)

- Instagram

- Facebook

- Twitter

- YouTube

- LinkedIn

- Podcasts

We see examples of this all the time. Ordinary people like you and us, including many other medical professionals, establish their authority in their niche simply by using platforms like these to communicate. This is how they create their own media.

It can be as simple as starting to do Instagram posts or YouTube videos. The key is to communicate with your target audience and provide valuable information. That's how you become the authority in that area.

A big mistake many make is to utilize too many media platforms at once. We recommend focusing on one at the start, and you can expand beyond that later if you wish.

Obviously, choosing a platform is the first part of the process, and you then need to fill your channel with content. That usually involves speaking, writing, or some combination of both, depending on what works best for you.

Believe it or not, there are patients who go to the local nutrition shop trying to get medical advice.

They would love to hear from an actual physician about other solutions for their health.

In order for them to know you exist, you have to do things which establish you as an authority.

We'll discuss the exact steps for doing that later in the chapter.

Evidence

Even when you are respected as an authority, people will want to see evidence that you are able to do what you claim.

The three main ways this can be done is through:

- Testimonials

- Case studies

- Endorsements

Testimonials allow people to see how you have worked with other people and the results they have achieved. A testimonial usually involves a previous patient talking about how they worked with you and their results.

Case studies are similar to testimonials. However, in this instance, it is you, the physician, giving an account of the patient's health issues. You relay the course of events in the patient's treatment and the clinical outcomes in the form of a story.

By telling a story, you make the process easy to understand and the potential client can identify with your patient and their journey.

Case studies are very useful whether or not you have testimonials.

Endorsements are when other experts recommend you to their audience.

It may be an endorsement of your skill from another medical professional, or it may be someone in another field introducing you to their audience.

Another form of endorsement is when one of your current patients recommends you to their family and friends.

All three of these may be governed by regulations depending on your specialty and your state. Be assured there are ways to utilize these approaches while staying within the guidelines.

Avoid This Big Mistake

In a moment, we'll talk about the exact steps you need to take to make this work. However, there is something we want to emphasize first.

We both feel one of our big mistakes was not getting out into the community sooner and connecting with other businesses and other healthcare providers who serviced our ideal clients. They were in need of hearing our message.

We started to see success when we could stand up in a room of strangers, talk to them about their health, give them another perspective, and then offer them an opportunity to work with us.

As you continue to communicate your message effectively, you start to find people coming up and saying, "Yes, I want what you're offering."

People are trusting the 20-year-old at the nutrition shop to give them medical advice when they would gladly come to see you for your expert opinion.

As we discussed earlier, in medicine, it's taught, "See one, do one, teach one." And you're only taught one way.

Dr. Henry started from ground zero with no clients and none to move over. Dr. Woods transitioned from an insurance-based to an independent, cash practice.

Our level of authority was fully intact, but we had no idea. Our perceived authority was minimal.

The main change to establish your authority requires a mindset shift and realization.

The fact is people are searching for answers, and they are trusting the 20-year-old at the nutrition shop to give them medical advice when they would gladly come to see you for your expert opinion.

Your Authority Action Plan – 5 Steps to Become the Authority in Your Market

Now let's talk about the exact steps you need to take in order to build your authority. There are five key steps you need to start with:

1. Choose your target market and ideal client

2. Construct your ideal media platform

3. Create educational content

4. Connect with your audience by speaking

5. Collect success stories and seek endorsements

Let's look more closely at what you need to do in each element.

1. Choose Your Target Market and Ideal Client

In the first part of this chapter, we discussed the idea of initially focusing on one area of expertise for marketing to attract your ideal client.

It's also unrealistic to think that you can deliver your services to the entire world. You need to focus on a particular market based on geography, your area of expertise and your ideal client for your practice. For example, you may only want to work with women with hormonal concerns or seniors with diabetes.

This decision process, known as choosing your niche, is one of the most important decisions you'll make in building your independent practice, as it will be a key factor in your success.

The choice involves two main elements

- Professional Expertise - this is about how you define your niche in terms of your medical expertise.

- People and Problems - this is about the people you serve and how you help them.

Professional Expertise

To some extent you will already have made choices about your field of expertise but remember you need to be as specific as possible. Here are some questions that will help guide your choice of niche.

- What specific area of medicine are you especially passionate about and can speak on without much thought?

- In what specific area of medicine have you seen patients get the best results from working with you?

- In what specific area of medicine have patients referred others to work with you based on their experience with you?

- What specific area of medicine have people asked you to come and speak to their organizations about?

- In what specific area of medicine do you attend at least one conference annually to improve your overall knowledge base to help patients?

- In what specific area of medicine have you done the most online searches and/or spoken to colleagues to get the information your patients need to improve their clinical outcomes?

People and Problems

When you choose your niche, you should be able to describe it in some detail, including information such as:

- Who you are serving

  o Gender, Age, Profession, Marital Status, Income

- What problem they have

  o What worries are keeping them up in the middle of the night?

- How you can reach this audience

  o Find out as much as you can about them. For example: where they hang out or shop, what they read, whether they are pet owners or travelers, what their hobbies are, what their religious beliefs and political affiliations are, whether they work-out.

Basically, you need to do some research to really get in their heads and find out how they think.

ACTION

Open a journal or a Google doc and write out the answers to the following questions.

1. What is your area of professional expertise?

2. What people will you serve and what problem will you help with?

3. How will you reach these people?

Example

Here is how Dr. Woods would answer these questions.

1. *What is your area of professional expertise? Obstetrics and Gynecology with an emphasis in bioidentical hormone replacement therapy.*

2. *What people will you serve and what problem will you help with? Women between the ages of 45-60 who are having issues with hot flashes, weight gain and decreased libido.*

3. *How will you reach these people? Through education-based marketing. Hosting free in-person seminars and online webinars. Speaking at facilities where these women convene (gym, yoga studio, spa, church).*

2. Construct Your Ideal Media Platform

When we talked about evangelism, we mentioned the many different platforms for getting your message across, such as your own blog, Facebook and Instagram.

Once you have decided on your niche, you need to establish which of the platforms is the best way to reach them.

This will first depend on your audience. Consider where they gather and how they consume information.

For example, some platforms may be more appropriate to certain niches, e.g.:

- Business Professionals – LinkedIn

- Millennials – Instagram

- Age 40-60 – Facebook

There is also a component of the platform decision that depends on you and your preferences.

For example, you will take into account your communication strengths and style. Maybe you are already a Facebook enthusiast and that works best for you. Maybe you love shooting videos and would be most happy on YouTube.

As we said earlier, the best approach is to choose one media platform to focus on initially and seek to master it rather than learning several and being average or poor in the way you use them.

ACTION

Answer the following question.

What social media platform are you going to focus on for getting your message across?

Example

Dr. Woods started by using Facebook ads to invite her ideal clients to a free in-person seminar. At the conclusion of the seminar, she invites the attendees to a paid consultation.

Dr. Woods also uses Facebook ads to offer a free report about "The 3 Secrets to Hormone Balance Every Woman Should Know." At the end of the report, there is an invitation to schedule a free "Ready to Feel Good Again" strategy call with Dr. Woods' team.

On the strategy call, the prospective client is then invited to schedule a paid consultation with Dr. Woods.

3. Create Educational Content

One of the important ways you let people know about your authority is through the educational content you produce.

Dr. Henry prefers to shoot pre-recorded and live videos to create content for her ideal audience. Dr. Henry also has a recorded webinar on diabetes that she markets with Facebook ads.

Once a potential patient sees the Facebook ad about diabetes, they are invited to watch a webinar called Reversing Diabetes Naturally.

The webinar provides educational content on Dr. Henry's approach to reversing diabetes naturally and is followed by an invitation to speak with her team to discuss any further questions.

Many people are overwhelmed by the idea of creating content. The truth is, it is much easier than most people think, and there is a wide range of resources and vendors that can help you.

There are really two ways you can create content, depending on what comes more naturally to you:

- Speak

- Write

For some people, speaking is easier than writing, so they prefer to create content by making videos or audio recordings.

Ways of using speaking to share your message include:

- Video

- Podcasts

- Webinars

- Live events

In doing this, you can then have the content transcribed so that it is also in written format. This allows you to repurpose your material, and your videos can then be turned into blogs, emails or newsletters.

Not everyone is a fluent and comfortable speaker. Some people are happier to sit down and write content such as:

- Blog posts

- Articles

- Special reports

As with spoken content, you can repurpose written material by turning it into audio and video. You can either record it yourself or hire someone to do that.

As you go forward, a book is a great way to exhibit your authority and expertise on a subject. Laying out your knowledge and the process by which you help people does not have to be a painful process, and there are many resources and experts available to help you write a book easily.

We've done it and you can, too!

The big advantage of having a book published is that you are automatically seen as an authority. This could result in invitations to speak at events or on podcasts or to do television, radio and other forms of media appearances.

A book could also help you connect with other business owners who provide services to your ideal client. Basically, it can be a means for a great referral base.

However, for most people writing a book is not the first step. We advise you to keep it simple initially and build from there.

If you don't have the time or inclination to write yourself, you can hire freelancers or staff to do it for you. Here are a few resources to check out.

Fiverr.com

Fiverr began with every service starting at $5 (a fiver). Some of the prices have gone up, but you can find social media help, blog writers, graphic designers, voice-overs, cartoon artists… and the list goes on!

Upwork.com

This site allows you to hire individuals to perform services or complete projects. If you choose Upwork, you may have an ongoing need for help versus a small project. There are workers from around the world who post their area of expertise. You can go on the site and find the person who is right for you and fits your budget.

GetLeverage.com

Leverage is a site that will address whatever issue you are having within your business and find the resources to support you. They do the heavy lifting. For instance, if you need help with creating educational content, the people at Leverage will interview and find writers for you. There is a monthly fee for Leverage services.

ACTION

Decide what educational content you will create.

Example

Dr. Henry wrote a book, The Unlimited You Detox, *and sends it to potential patients as part of her authority builder.*

Dr. Woods uses a glossy, full-color 10-page report about "The 3 Secrets to Hormone Balance Every Woman Should Know." Her report is mailed out to every client who schedules a consultation.

4. Connect to Audiences by Speaking

There is no doubt that one of the best ways to establish your authority and reach out to the right audience is by speaking to groups – large and small.

It doesn't have to be an audience of thousands. The best audience of all can be half a dozen people in your office who have come along because they are interested in what you offer.

That's why one of the most important aspects of speaking is not what you say but who is in your audience.

Of course, you may be somewhat apprehensive – most people are in the beginning. That's why it's so rewarding for those who are willing to do it. So, don't be intimidated by this idea of public speaking.

You have a vast bank of knowledge, and any client or prospective client would be eager to learn from you. Stop and think about it. You talk to your patients every day in the office about health-related issues.

Or how about when you are at a family or friends get together and a medical question comes up? Who do they turn to for the expert opinion? Even if there are people in the room who are health savvy, where do they go to get the final word? YOU! Because you are the EXPERT.

When you think about it, it is quite easy to discuss a topic that you are totally comfortable and familiar with.

Those topics flow from you like you were born knowing it. Your knowledge is so valuable though you may not see that because it comes so easy to you.

If you are not yet comfortable with doing live talks, or these don't fit in well with your schedule, then do a webinar. You can pre-record this in advance or at least present it to a small audience.

There really is no excuse not to deliver your message to your ideal client. It boils down to making it as easy as possible for yourself. One way to do that is to create one signature talk or a standard presentation, which covers the key information you need to get across and how you can help your ideal client.

By the way, a great advantage of speaking to audiences is that you get to hear from them, understand their concerns and develop greater empathy for them.

As with all of these steps, the key is to start with a small step, build your confidence, get some success and grow from there.

ACTION

1. Decide the content of your core presentation.

2. Identify an audience to whom you can deliver your talk.

Example

For example, Dr. Henry's talks have been focused on reversing diabetes naturally and have been delivered via live talks and both live and pre-recorded webinars.

5. Collect Success Stories and Seek Endorsements

Another one of the keys to establishing your authority is providing the success stories of patients who know the results you can deliver through testimonials, case studies and endorsements.

The key is that you need to have a system in place to collect these great patient outcomes.

For testimonials, one thing you can do is determine at what time during the course of working with a client they feel most positive.

For example, if all of your patients are raving about how good they feel at their two-month follow-up visit, you should routinely ask everyone for a testimonial.

To systematize this process, you can put a reminder on the chart or on their appointment slot, ASK FOR TESTIMONIAL, at the two-month follow-up visit.

Have your receptionist or assistant add this note every time a two-month visit is scheduled.

You could use this simple script to ask for the testimonial:

"I'm so excited that you are doing well. I would love to share your success story so that others understand that it is possible for them to feel great as well.

It is my goal to help as many people as possible. But I need help spreading the word.

Would you be willing to share your success story? May we shoot a quick video or would you prefer to do it in writing?"

For case studies, think about some examples that you could share with prospective clients that show how your system works.

You also want to get endorsements from people who are already well known to your target audience.

ACTION

1. Review what testimonials you currently have.

2. Put in place a process for collecting testimonials consistently.

3. Identify some case studies that you have or could develop.

4. Identify key influencers that could endorse you and introduce you to their audiences.

Example

For example, Dr. Woods was invited to speak at a gym by one of her patients who is doing extremely well and has been a long-time advocate of her practice.

With an intimate group of 16 women, Dr. Woods presented her signature talk on hormones, answered questions, and signed up eight women for a paid consultation. That was without any Facebook ads or paid marketing.

Creating an Action Plan

Now that you have identified the key actions needed, you need to turn them into an action plan.

First, you have to identify the task you want to complete, e.g., set up a Facebook page.

Then work out the exact steps needed to make that happen.

Next, allocate the responsibility for the next steps and the dates they need to be completed by.

Finally, take the first step and start making it happen.

We recommend that you map out your marketing plan at least three months ahead. But don't overcomplicate it. You can't do everything at once. What matters is getting started and making continual improvement.

Don't Hold Back

Patients need to see and hear that you are the expert. You are an authority in your area. No more modesty. No more being in the background.

Think about all the money you spent getting your education. All the conferences you have attended. The platforms and panels you have participated on.

Some of you have even been on national TV, spoken on podcasts, and have been featured in local newspapers, TV and radio.

This is nothing to speak lightly of. This is how you establish your authority. Current clients, prospective patients, and your colleagues want to hear from you, and they truly value your opinion.

It's time to step into and own your authority. So, please drop the modesty. It doesn't serve anyone.

It's now time to claim your expert status. You have worked hard, and now it's time to share it with those outside of your immediate circle.

Chapter 7: Value – How to Make Sure Your Patients are Happy to See You Without Using Their Insurance

If you're going to build a successful independent practice, you need to be able to convince a steady stream of patients to see you without using their insurance.

And if you are going to achieve the lifestyle that you want, you need to make sure you deliver a high-quality experience and help patients achieve great transformational outcomes.

When these goals are met, your patients will be more than happy to invest in your premium programs.

The Value Formula

The concept of value revolves around three elements:

- **Self-Worth:** How you feel about what you are charging

- **Perceived Value:** How much it is worth to the patient

- **Received Value:** How the person feels about paying the price after the experience

So, the Physician Value Formula is:

$$SW \times PV \times RV = Total\ Value$$

Let's start by talking about what each of these means and then we'll look at how to maximize them.

#1: Self-Worth

As physicians, we are often uncomfortable with the subject of money, and that holds us back in various ways.

First, we don't like to talk about money or spend much time thinking about it. If we are employed, we take the salary and leave the money issues to someone else. Even in our own practices, we typically leave someone else to handle all the negotiation with insurance companies about reimbursements.

As physicians, we often have the idea in our minds that talking about money downgrades us. We're supposed to be altruistic and focus on helping people and improving their health.

But to succeed in an independent practice, you have to be more conscious of financial issues and more involved in them.

When you are not fully aware of the financial health and status of your practice, you risk losing opportunities for improvement and you increase the risk of a failed business.

While helping others is the most common reason why a person chooses the field of medicine, you cannot help anyone if you don't run your business wisely.

Thinking positively about money is also vital if you are to achieve the kind of lifestyle you want for yourself and your family. The money won't flow if you don't pay it due attention.

One of the challenges with determining self-worth is getting a clear understanding of what you are really worth.

If you apply for an employed position and are offering standard services, it's usually easy to get a comparison.

Many of us have searched the internet for the industry standards for compensation in our particular area based on our years of experience. This is how many physicians determine how much they should be compensated.

However, it's important to remember that this is the average and is not always based on the most accurate information. If most physicians are undervaluing their services, why would you want to compare yourself to those standards? Perhaps you should aim higher and compare yourself to something different.

> *You will not be able to help anyone if you don't run your business wisely.*

For example, we hear about the great wealth being earned by business executives and by sports and film stars.

Yet physicians are saving lives and helping to improve people's quality of life while making only cents on the dollar.

We are not implying physicians should be paid the same as athletes, film stars, or corporate leaders, but we will press the issue of you as a physician being paid what you are worth. The fact is, we are getting paid less and less.

Just stop and think. When was the last time someone in the healthcare field sat down with you and said, "You are worth so much more?"

Well, let's say it right here and now.

You Are Worth So Much More.

Yes, we know you know you are valued as a person by your family, friends and colleagues. But honestly, when was the last time you questioned the amount that gets deposited in the bank by your employer/insurance company or bill collecting service?

For too long as physicians, we have not questioned what we are being paid.

When you think about your value, there are several things you need to take into account.

One of these is reflecting on the fees charged by our employers or insurance companies for what we deliver. As we often say, if you are being paid $100, say, for a specific service, how much is that generating for the hospital or insurance company – three, four, five times that amount?

Another thing to consider is what is the value of what you deliver to the patient in relation to other things they will spend money on, such as leisure and vacations. We'll talk more about that in a moment.

Most of us have invested hundreds of thousands of dollars to get where we are.

Another factor to consider as it relates to the value you provide is the amount you have invested to develop your expertise.

Most of us have invested hundreds of thousands of dollars to get where we are and consistently educate ourselves to remain current with information to help patients on a daily basis. That's truly a class act.

The fact is you are a highly educated access point for patients who are trying to improve their health.

Are you getting the picture? As you reassess your situation and look to build or consider starting an independent practice, it's important you allocate some time to evaluate your situation and your worth. It's time to own your worth!

To maximize your self-worth, you need to change your mindset about money.

In a moment, we'll talk about some steps you can take to do that.

#2: Perceived Value

The next aspect of value that's important is understanding what something is worth to someone.

Value can be defined in numerous ways. For this purpose, we define value as: "To have a high opinion of; the extent to which a service is perceived by a patient to meet his or her need which is determined by the patient's willingness to pay for the service."

There is a famous story of a rich factory owner who had an urgent problem with his heating system that was preventing the factory from operating and it was costing thousands of dollars per day. He called in an engineer who took a look around the factory and then tapped on one of the pipes and fixed the problem.

Despite what the problem had been costing him, the factory owner was horrified when he received an invoice for the repairs at a cost of $1,000. He argued, "That's outrageous. You were here less than an hour." So, the engineer revised his invoice to say, "Attending factory to repair heating system – $100. For knowing where to tap – $900."

The factory owner could not argue with that.

The key lesson is that the way you present costs is important so that people see the true value of what they are getting.

To look at it in another way, think back to a gift you may have received. It may have been something considered to be nice, but it wasn't what you really wanted. Thus, it just sat on the shelf, collected dust, was moved to the back of the closet, and eventually placed in the giveaway pile. If your dear mother-in-law knew what you had done to that expensive sweater she bought you!

The fact is it just didn't mean that much to you because it wasn't something you valued. In addition, it's something that didn't cost you anything.

The value we ascribe to something is often a reflection of what we paid for it. People generally don't value things that are free or cheap.

When you underprice your services, it's just like that expensive sweater being thrown in the giveaway box.

Yet you are still surprised by how many do not take you up on these severely discounted offerings. You are also frustrated by how many do not get results because of their lack of compliance.

This should NOT be surprising at all. Here is a little-known secret amongst physicians...

People value what they pay for, and they are more likely to place time and energy into getting results when they have more skin in the game.

Often the best clients are those who are willing to pay a bit more. But you need to take steps to show them that what you are offering is worth so much more than the investment you are proposing.

To do that, and in order to maximize the perceived value, you need to create and present a powerful offer. We'll talk about how to do that in a moment.

#3: Received Value

At this point, we can agree your services and the transformation you bring about is highly valuable.

But let's be upfront with one another. Value can be defined in numerous ways. To deliver value, we need to make sure that the whole experience is one that makes the patient feel their investment will be worthwhile and that they still feel the same way afterwards.

As part of this, it is important that your patients realize they are working with an authority in medicine who is highly sought after.

That alone is not enough.

To raise your patient's experience level and their received value, we suggest using what we call the WOW factor.

Now, you may be thinking, "What's this WOW factor?" This is merely the things we do to create value for our clients. We are shifting the value focus from us to the patient. The patient needs to see the true value in you and your services.

By the way, it's important as you read this that you continue to keep an open mind on how this all works. We are not suggesting unnecessary tricks and gimmicks.

This is a systematic approach that will help give you back time, increase your income and expand your impact.

The overall process is designed to help patients select you and your services based on your ability to meet their health concerns.

As part of that, at some point, you will need to say something along the lines of "This is my fee so pay me!"

We advise you NOT to say it in those exact words, but you should have this thought in mind, "This is the value of my services, and I know I'm worth it."

> *The patient needs to see the true value in you and your services.*

A key point to bear in mind is that not everyone will see that value, and that is ok. Be assured that, with the right message and following the formula we outline, you will connect with the right people who will be more than happy to pay you what you're worth.

We will show you how to demonstrate value through your authority, celebrity factor, and expert status, all of which contribute to the WOW factor.

The right patients will understand and appreciate your expertise and will be ready to move forward and work with you and your team.

Enhancing Value

The elements above make up the Value Formula so to maximize the value, we need to increase each element as much as possible.

Another way of describing our Value Formula is:

$$\textit{Mindset x Offer x Experience = Total Value}$$

So, let's look at how to maximize each.

#1: Maximizing Self-Worth – Changing the Money Mindset

One of the biggest hurdles for physicians who we work with is the fear of, "Will people pay x amount for my services?"

When we started out, we were fearful at first to ask for a payment at all.

We weren't sure if someone who had insurance would even pay for a service we offered.

And to add insult to injury, even your family, friends and colleagues will ask the same thing, "Do you REALLY think someone will pay that much?"

These questions and doubts can really be a blow to your confidence about your entire business model.

But we're here to say, "Don't be discouraged!"

Just keep your mind focused on the idea that what you are providing is of great value, and you don't need every prospect you encounter to become your client.

You only need to connect with the RIGHT clients.

Those are the ones who:

- Understand what you do

- See the value of what you offer

- Are willing to invest in the transformation you can help them achieve

It's just that simple. As we mentioned earlier, one of the ways to get over the money mindset hurdle is stopping to think about this one thing. PEOPLE WILL PAY FOR WHAT THEY VALUE.

Just think of some of the things your patients will spend money on:

- Cell phones and other tech gadgets

- Car costs

- Vacations

- Home remodeling

- Going out to eat

- Daily coffee at the local cafe

Think even about the health-related things people spend money on:

- Nutritional Supplements

- Aesthetic services (Botox), laser hair and facial treatments

- Online programs from health gurus

- Exercise equipment

- Workout DVDs and subscriptions

- Gym memberships

The truth is, people are paying for health and wellness related things all the time without the help of their insurance.

Money mindset fears, or the scarcity mentality, is quite common. The scarcity mindset is the idea that there is not enough money in the world. Or that your success will take away from someone else's success.

A better way to look at this is to recognize that the "pie" is really infinite. You charging what you are worth will not cause a detriment to anybody. In fact, those who do invest in your program will be most rewarded.

As we mentioned earlier, those who invest in their health will get better outcomes because they will take your recommendations and your program that much more seriously. Exactly because they don't want to waste the investment they made.

If you are going to be a **Physician Unleashed**, you have to step outside the box of common thinking. Get rid of the herd mentality and being satisfied with doing and thinking like the masses.

To truly be **unleashed**, it only requires you to see what's going on in society.

People pay for things they want. They pay for what they value. And they're paying for health and wellness all the time.

Your Ideal Patient Will Pay More

What helped us make the money mindset shift from being fearful of asking for payment to realizing this was just an important part of how we help patients was this idea of selling health.

Those who pay and, in fact, those who pay more are more invested in making change.

For example, if you buy a $5 tank top at Old Navy and it rips, that's not such a big deal. However, if you purchase a $200 name brand shirt and it gets torn, you are more likely to be bothered.

Furthermore, every time you wear the $200 shirt, you're more likely to take extra care NOT to cause any damage to it.

In the same way, a financial investment in health makes a difference.

Patients usually place more time and effort into the recommended treatment plan if they have made a significant investment.

For example, Dr. Woods learned this lesson when she first started an independent practice in 2013 and was focused on weight loss. Patients could see her for $115 per month and get their prescription refilled.

Most of those patients did so-so. It was a lot of losing and gaining the same three to five pounds. There was a rare one in the bunch who actually lost a significant amount of weight and kept it off.

Those who invest in their health will get better outcomes because they will take your recommendations and your program that much more seriously.

In contrast, when she started offering more comprehensive programs, ranging from $2,000-$10,000, these patients were much more compliant and committed to the process. One patient who purchased one of these premium programs lost 27 pounds in just three months and wrote a glowing review about it on Google.

No doubt you can better understand why a higher investment results in better outcomes. If you invest several thousand dollars on a wellness program, you will be much more likely to follow the program versus spending $115 per month. The low monthly fee was of little value.

To fully embrace this idea of value, you have to look at it this way. You are actually helping your patients do better by requiring them to make a substantial investment in their health.

The more they are invested, emotionally and financially, the more likely they are to be committed and compliant.

This type of dedication most often leads to obtainable and sustainable results.

In summary, focus on the change you make in people's lives, not some external idea of what it should cost.

> **ACTION: Change Your Money Mindset**
>
> 1. Add up the total amount you have invested in your medical education over the years.
>
> 2. List the ways that a patient benefits from working with you and estimate how much each element could be worth to them.
>
> 3. Consider other things that people happily buy for a similar value.
>
> 4. List some of the things people buy where price is not a factor.

#2: Maximizing Perceived Value – Creating and Selling a Package

The next element is demonstrating value to the patient. The steps involved in this are:

1. Show the result they could expect

2. Shape the offer to suit their situation

3. Set the price that will deliver value and profit

4. Sell the value to make it easy to buy

Step #1: Show the result they could expect

There are plenty of people who have a big enough pain point who will be looking for your services. By pain point, we mean what is keeping them up at night? What is the reason they sought you out in the first place? What is causing them such havoc that they don't care whether or not you take insurance?

Not every client is right for you. And you need to get used to the idea that not every person you offer your services to will be ready to jump on board. This is completely normal.

But this is also different from the insurance world where everyone who walks through the door is "your patient." Understand those most suited for an independent physician's practice are those who have reached a tipping point.

Most individuals are accustomed to their insurance and the services provided. After addressing and re-addressing the same issues with their traditional doctor, there comes a point when they realize they're not getting results. They say to themselves, "Something's not right."

There is a small subset of those who are not getting results from what their insurance provides who will step outside the box. They recognize their health is falling apart, and they decide "I have to do something. I don't care what it costs."

This group will make up most of your ideal clients. They have reached the tipping point where insurance coverage is no longer an issue.

A new client that started recently said, "I will pay anything to not feel this way because everybody keeps telling me I need to go on antidepressants." She had reached her tipping point.

> *There's a subset of patients who have a big pain point and have reached their tipping point and are ready to pay outside of their insurance.*

It's like when your patient gets sick and tired of being sick and tired or she gets tired of not getting answers or getting told that "there's nothing wrong. You're absolutely normal." Or she gets tired of hearing, "Let me put you on another prescription medication."

For some people, they have to reach that point, or they've watched a family member or a close friend get to a particular point in their health. They may be thinking, "I don't want to go that route. The traditional system is not working, so I have to do something different."

Most people think all of their health issues should be covered by their health insurance. Most doctors also would like to believe health insurance covers the majority of healthcare. But there's a subset of patients who have a big pain point. They have reached their tipping point, and they're ready to pay outside of their insurance.

Patients willingly pay for health coaches, acupuncturists and many other alternative therapies.

When it comes to paying a medical doctor, there is an unfortunate hesitation because of the misconception that everything should be covered by health insurance.

The key to move past this reluctance is to demonstrate exactly the result they can expect.

What you need to be able to do is paint a picture of what life will be like for them after they have followed your program.

The ways you can do this include:

- Case studies of other people who have followed your program

- Description of how their symptoms could change

- Present success stories of patients with similar health concerns

ACTION

What can you do to demonstrate the results your patients could achieve?

Step #2: Shape the offer to suit their situation

One of the key elements of demonstrating value is the personalized program you put together that your potential patient can choose to buy.

You need to give them a clearly written document with the details of the program that addresses their health concerns.

Our preferred method of putting together an offer is to create a program or package in which the services are bundled.

The idea behind this is that a bundled program or package emphasizes the overall range and value of what you are offering.

You put this together and offer it as one bundled price. This ensures they can make one decision and commit to all of the stages involved rather than having to make lots of individual choices.

Putting together this sort of program or package that delivers value is not something they taught us in medical school. We learned how to create a valuable program by observing others in different fields, implementing our ideas and adapting the offer through trial and error based on what worked.

We showed our prospective clients the value in the systems and methods we used and learned to demonstrate how our systems were superior to the other things they had tried.

It was very important to relate to patients on a personal level and tell them, "I hear you, and I will partner with you on this journey to better health." But we also needed to have a specific offer that they could look at and make a decision about.

In creating a package, you have to truly identify what the person in front of you really needs to do in order to get to their best level of health.

We do not make any health outcome promises, only that we will support them 100% along the way and help them identify the areas of their health that need to be improved.

As you get feedback, you will make changes. For example, Dr. Henry streamlined one of her programs from six months down to four months. She found people wanted to get better as soon as possible, and they were able to achieve success in a shorter period of time.

Keys Elements to a High-Value Program

The basic formulas that physicians can follow as they start to piece together their programs include:

- Number of visits

- Specialty tests

- Personalized treatment plans

- Other elements (visits with health coach or nutritionists, supplements or supplement discounts)

It is important to realize that the initial investment of the patient is time and energy. Maintaining interest and excitement is in the hands of the physician and their team.

The reason why programs work is because the client is committed to the entire process required for success: visits, specialty tests and a commitment to the transformation process.

When it comes to visits, we strongly suggest avoiding the common practice among physicians of offering a visit by visit approach, i.e., when your client pays for one visit at a time.

We have found the visit by visit approach reduces compliance, increases no-show rates and can hinder your patients' commitment to make lasting changes with their health.

On the other hand, if someone has prepaid or purchased a block of visits, they are more likely to return because they have already invested.

They are also more likely to do the work required because they have built-in accountability.

They know they will have a check-in with you and your team soon and will need to give a report of their progress.

With a bundled program, there are fewer no-shows. You will be able to spend more time with each patient and get paid what you're worth.

For the business, with pay as you go programs, there is less predictable cash flow and there is a lower perceived value. The business and the patient are adversely affected.

This formula is so powerful that once the patients start to get results as it relates to their health concerns, many want to continue to work with you.

The key to success with a bundled program is to recognize the patient's concerns and have an achievable solution with a clear path that is specific to each person with built-in accountability.

Specialty tests are another key component. Some of the common specialty tests we order include: a comprehensive DNA PCR-based stool test, food sensitivity testing and cortisol.

The results of these tests allow the program to be tailored to the individual based on their presenting initial concerns.

For additional services, an essential piece that is often missed in physician's offices is nutritional counseling.

Because there is so much confusion regarding the impact of food on the body, we believe counseling on nutrition must be included in the design of the patient's program.

Whether this counseling is provided by a physician, nutritionist, or health coach, someone needs to spend some significant time with the patient talking about food.

These meetings are not only about food choices but how to design their life around these new life habits.

There are many discussions about the obstacles patients face as they embark on their health journey. We address how to handle spouses and children that may not support the changes and who may not be keen on changing their diet.

To put it all together, a common diabetes program consists of 12 visits over six months.

The program includes visits with the physician, nutritional counseling, exercise recommendations and specialty labs.

The package allows the patient to make a one-time investment in the program, and it removes any insurance-based constraint, allowing the physician to spend more time and give the best care.

Now, it goes without saying, each program needs to be tweaked based on what health concerns are presented to you. But this is easy because you have a foundational formula.

Remember, stick with this basic formula, and you will see great success.

ACTION

Next step is to design the contents of your own program:

1. What number of visits will you include?

2. What specialty tests will you provide?

3. What will the personalized treatment plans include?

4. What other elements will you offer?

As you design your program, bear in mind that you may offer some variations to your program to cover different types of patient needs. But try to develop a program that works for most people and have as few variations to it as possible.

Step #3: Set the price that will deliver value and profit

The next important decision is working out what price you will charge for your program.

In doing this, you have to take into account what it costs you to deliver the service, including the costs of marketing plus a decent profit margin.

So, you need to start by listing out all the costs involved. In the example we used previously, the costs might be:

- Specialty Tests

- Staffing Costs

- Nutritionist or Health Coach Costs

- Supplements

- Your Hourly Rate

- Operational Costs (rent, utilities, etc.)

On top of that, you need to add in a marketing allowance. Marketing dollars may be spent on Facebook ads, direct mail pieces, and dinners (if doing dinner talks). The cost of your marketing team also needs to be considered.

Finally, you will arrive at an estimate of the cost. To set the price, you need to decide what profit margin you want to make, and then you set the final price.

Remember the key is to arrive at an appropriate price. It's not to make it as cheap as possible.

As we said, people will value what they put their money into. So, we could offer the same program for $50 or $5,000. The person who pays $5,000 is more likely do better.

They have more of a stake in their success than someone paying very little.

In principle, it will also be much easier for you to make one $5,000 sale than 100 sales at $50. However, you have to come up with a price that will work for enough of the right prospective patients.

When Dr. Woods started out, she was offering a program that was $99 a month. But she quickly realized she could help more people with a more expensive program.

You may have to test different prices and perhaps offer some different options to work out what is best.

For example, you could offer silver, gold and platinum options at different prices with varying elements included to appeal to different people.

You will also have to consider whether you want to offer financing or payment terms.

A tip to bear in mind when setting your prices is that things are often more expensive than you realize, and it is important to consider all expenses that might need to be included when you are setting your program fees.

As we discussed under mindset, make sure you charge what you are worth.

We learned this early on while sitting in a room listening to health coaches, dieticians, chiropractors and acupuncturists.

It was shocking to discover they were all charging more than us.

When we told them our rates, they all looked back at us like, "What's wrong with you? You immediately have credibility. We have to prove ourselves. As medical doctors, you don't."

The fact is, of all the people in the healthcare space, you, the medical doctor, are at the top of the trust food chain.

However, most physicians are not actively trying to get their message out to the public like other healthcare practitioners.

The problem is physicians generally don't know much about marketing or how to get their message to the public because most of us have never had to do that. We thought we just needed to put up our sign "Doctor Here," and the patients would roll in.

As she started her practice, Dr. Henry was speaking to a chiropractor at a conference. That chiropractor's rates were three to four times more, and she told Dr. Henry, "If you don't change things around, you're going to be broke. You've got to change."

So, make sure you are charging enough for the transformation you will deliver.

For us, a big mistake was not charging what we were worth sooner.

ACTION

Determine the direct costs for the program(s) you plan to offer while also considering all of your indirect costs (overhead expenses) required to run your business.

Add your desired profit margin to the direct and indirect costs, and the total of these two will be the price of your program.

Examples of indirect costs are rent, staffing, utilities, internet, phone and marketing.

Direct cost examples are the prices of specialty tests and supplements.

Step #4: Sell the value to make it easy to buy

To make this whole process work, you have to be ready to sell your program.

Here it's important to bear in mind that running an independent practice means you are not just a doctor. You are in the business of sales. You are selling health.

As we said earlier in the book, many physicians are uncomfortable with the idea of selling.

This partly goes back to the entitlement mentality. Physicians think they do not have to work to get patients through the door.

Some physicians think of sales as being sleazy. They think it goes against where their interest should lie, which is with the greater good of the patient.

However, we need to recognize that all selling isn't bad. Sales is a natural part of our transaction of services and data. People generally like to buy things.

Our hesitation about sales may be a reflection of the fact that it's something we as physicians typically have not had to do. Yet, like most things, it's a lot easier when you know what needs to be done.

Getting good at sales is partly about changing the way you think about it.

It's also about having the right tools and processes to make it easy. We'll look at how you can improve in both of these areas.

<u>The Mindset of Selling</u>

It's important to remember that what we are selling here is health. If we can convince someone to buy what we are offering, we are helping the patient get better, so we're doing them a good service.

Many times, what we have to do is explain the options to people and help them to see the value. In some cases, showing value is about being very honest with the person about their situation and what is required to really change.

This direct approach may be viewed as blunt to some of you. But that may be what is required to snap your client into taking action.

For example, a recent conversation with a prospective patient went like this: "This is what you need. This is where your health is declining. Either you're going to eat rice and cookies and stay on your medication, or stop eating those things and come off of it. Make a choice."

In being clear and direct about your patient's current health status, you are acting as the trusted physician authority.

You are telling them what they need to do, and many will respond positively. You then need to present the options to them on how they can move forward.

Being willing to push and challenge your patients a bit actually shows them that you care. And that is priceless. Being direct while showing empathy is a great way to show value.

Sales doesn't have to be a nasty word. It is simply an exchange. Something of value is given in return for something of value received.

The Tools of Selling

In order to present program options to your prospective patient, you need to have the right tools in place. A great tool is one that allows you to get your message across through education-based marketing followed by an offer to work with you.

One signature presentation is an example of a selling tool. A signature presentation is a PowerPoint presentation on a hot topic of interest to your potential client. It is one that you can use over and over again. Either in a live event, as a live webinar or as a pre-recorded webinar.

Another example of a selling tool is a free report about a topic of interest to your ideal client.

To check out Dr. Woods' free report about hormones, visit drwoodswellness.com/guide.

In addition, you need a step-by-step patient acquisition process to move a person from a potential client to a paying client.

To make sure this process produces predictable and reliable results, you may want to script out this process and the conversations related to each step.

When done correctly, the patient acquisition process will result in a new client who has excitedly decided to purchase a program in order to work with you, the trusted authority.

Here is an example of how the patient acquisition process could work for your business.

- Your potential client would first come to know of you through a free report or a pre-recorded webinar available on your website.

- In order for them to view the report or watch the webinar, they must provide their name and email address.

- At the end of the free report and webinar, there is a "call to action." This is a marketing term which means you invite the potential client to take an action step, which will lead them closer to making a decision to work with you.

- Your call to action is an invitation to schedule a free brief phone call. We call this phone call a strategy call.

- If the potential client does not immediately schedule a strategy call after reading your report or watching your webinar, you follow-up with an email inviting them again to schedule the strategy call.

- Your goal on the strategy call is to review their health challenges and determine if they are ready to move forward with an in-office consultation.

- During the consultation, you will have discussed their health concerns and truly heard what is preventing them from living their best life. At the conclusion of the consultation, you will make a recommendation regarding which program you think is the best fit.

The two of you have now established a plan of action to reach their health goals.

Without any hesitation, this once prospective patient is now ready to take action with you and your team to start their health transformation.

Our typical consultation is approximately one hour. With the typical time restraints removed, the doctor is able to fully connect beyond the diagnosis, and the patient has felt heard and understands the next steps in their health journey.

Now that's healthcare at its best – a true doctor-patient relationship!

Ethical Obligation and Fair Exchange

Of course, you should always sell health ethically and with a high moral obligation.

With the level of chronic disease and death in America and the rising rates around the world, you need to make every effort to help as many people as you can.

You also need to earn a decent living and feel good about not only what you are doing but also how you are being compensated for the services you provide.

That means fair exchange is important. Think back to one of those difficult patients you have had to deal with in the past.

They take up tons of time in your office, and they don't comply with your recommendations. Then they return, seemingly upset with you, because they are no better.

How many times have you said under your breath as you left the room or complained to your colleagues: "I don't get paid enough to deal with this nonsense!"

That is an unfair exchange.

You have given the value of your time and your attention, not to mention the expertise of your specialty.

In return, you received a $20 co-pay, and you will have to wait anywhere from two weeks to 90 days to receive the other small portion of pay the insurance company reimburses you.

That is ridiculous, and you DON'T get paid enough to deal with that! Especially when you have a waiting room full of patients to see, you are running behind, and you missed lunch.

Now, just imagine if your entire schedule for the day had only five people. You have 30-60 minutes allotted for each patient.

This same patient comes in, and instead of the quick exchange and you being on edge about how behind you will be, you sit down, put your laptop aside, and look your patient in the eye.

You give her some truth about her situation in a caring, empathetic manner.

Now she believes you do care about her and you're not just trying to rush her out of the room. She admits to herself and to you that you are right and she needs to make some changes soon or her health will continue to decline.

You walk away thinking, "I think she heard me, and I believe she's going to do better."

She walks away thinking, "My doctor really cares about me."

ACTION

1. Mindset: How can you revise the way you think about sales to reduce your worry?

2. Tools: What presentations or scripts can you develop to simplify the sales process?

#3: Maximizing Received Value – Delivering a "WOW" Experience

Now that you believe you are worth the fees you are charging and you have created and presented a valuable offer at the right price, is your practice set up for success?

You may have started off well. But if you do not do something to stand out from other physicians, you may not reach your full potential. You have to go beyond the basics and stand out from the crowd.

To be truly successful, you need to go beyond what people expect and deliver what we call the WOW experience.

There are three elements to this:

- Before they sign up for your program

- During the time in your program

- After the program is complete

Here's the reason we call it a WOW experience. If you are successful at each stage, they are:

- Willing to give you a try

- Over the moon with the program

- Won over to your practice and ready to recommend you to others

Let's look at each of these elements.

Before they sign up for your program

Many of your potential new clients have probably never have heard of you and don't know much about you before the first interaction with you.

They will have to discover your authority and expertise quickly and learn about how they can benefit from your services.

We have to start building the WOW experience right from the first interaction, and the steps in this process have to be carefully designed. Let's say someone starts by visiting your website. Here's how the process might develop:

- In exchange for giving you their email address, you send them a downloadable blueprint such as, "Dr. Smith's Top 6 Shocking Facts Every Woman Should Know about Hormones."

- The same day the prospective patient receives an email with a 45-second video thanking them for downloading the blueprint and offering them the opportunity to jump on a free 15-minute phone call with one of your clinical advisors.

- The next day the patient receives a call from your staff acknowledging their download of the blueprint and offering them a phone call and also a hard copy of your newest report.

- Later you may send a larger "shock and awe" package with a video and more detailed information for those who schedule a paid consultation. This would be sent out before their appointment. A shock and awe package might include: your book, a glossy full-color report, a small gift and a letter signed by you stating you are excited to meet them.

We'll talk more about this process in the next chapter, but the key here is that you are starting a WOW experience from the very beginning. This is not just a one-time, transactional sales process. You are developing a relationship with your potential client.

The goal is to pre-sell them before the paid consultation. We provide helpful information. It includes testimonials. The goal is to show up in the minds of your clients like nobody else. What other doctor has sent them videos and packages in the mail all about their health concerns? Get them excited to meet you before they even sit down with you.

During the time in your program

The next step in the process is creating a WOW experience for the potential client from the moment they enter into your system. For example, when you walk into our offices:

- There's a tea cart

- Essential oils are diffusing

- Soft music is playing in the background

This creates an atmosphere where the patient understands they are getting something that is unique, special and high quality. These added features create an enjoyable and memorable experience.

After the program is complete

The end of the program should not be the end of the experience. This should be the time when people are most likely to recommend you to other potential patients.

In fact, if they have bought from you once before, there is an increased likelihood they will buy from you again. And yes, that is a good thing. Think about what else you can offer.

We both have maintenance/membership programs, which allow patients to maintain the success they have experienced while being in our program.

Patients are more likely to stay with doctors they know, like, trust, and get results from.

You need to make the overall experience for your prospective patient feel worthwhile.

ACTION

Design the elements you will add to create a WOW experience.

1. Before they sign up for your program

2. During the time in your program

3. After the program is complete

Chapter 8: Systems – Attracting a Steady Stream of Clients and Building Your Practice Easily

To become a Physician Unleashed, you not only need to have a steady stream of ideal clients who buy repeatedly and refer, but you also need to have a practice that operates smoothly, allowing you maximum time with your patients.

The key to achieving those objectives is to have effective systems in place.

You can't rely on random acts of marketing and implementation and expect to get consistent results in either patient flow or patient satisfaction.

The idea of systems is common in science and medicine, and it's similar in business. You want to have results that are predictable and repeatable based on the actions you take in different situations.

Repeated Success

We have discovered focusing on certain key systems will set your practice up for repeated phenomenal success.

We talked earlier about how the problem for many physicians is the Revenue Roller Coaster.

This is usually the result of poor systems and can be avoided by putting good systems in place.

Systems should be in place for every aspect of your practice, starting before the very first time a potential patient encounters you (via website, Facebook, live presentations or webinars) all the way through to becoming a paying client.

These systems should also be utilized to foster a relationship with your patient that lasts for many years. That means you need a variety of systems, including:

- Lead Generation and Conversion

- Onboarding of New Patients

- Follow-up Appointments

- Obtaining Patient Testimonials

- Requesting Referrals from Existing Patients

- Patient Retention and Reactivation

We've found the better our systems are, the more solid the foundation is for our businesses.

The big mistake we made was not understanding the value of systems in the beginning and not getting them started sooner.

As with most things in business, you won't have perfect systems from the start. The key is to realize their importance and to start developing them in key areas.

You will keep improving these systems, and when you see how well they work, you will expand the use of systems in as many areas of your practice as possible.

In this chapter, we'll focus on what you need to do to set up one of the most important systems in your practice – the Lead Generation and Conversion System. This will keep your business growing.

Lead Generation and Conversion System

One of the most vital systems that will support the success of your practice is the one that delivers you a steady stream of potential patients that are ready to consider signing up for your program.

An effective system will deliver the new patients you need at minimum cost and with as little involvement by you in the process as possible.

We call this process Lead Generation and Conversion:

- A lead is a potential patient or client who has expressed an interest in your services but has not yet signed up to work with you.

- Lead generation is the process you use to garner the attention of those who may be interested in your services.

- Conversion is the process you use to turn some of those leads into paying patients.

Having a system like this ensures you do not waste your time with random acts of selling and marketing. You want to spend the time and dollars you commit to marketing on effective strategies you can measure.

This is not the time to be shooting darts in the sky, hoping they will land somewhere. That includes things like paying a social media company to get you more Likes on your Facebook page. A Like will never put a dollar in your bank account.

Here are the key elements and steps of the Lead Generation and Conversion System.

- Step #1: Target your ideal patients

- Step #2: Attract their attention

- Step #3: Capture their contact details

- Step #4: Build trust with them

- Step #5: Convert them to patients

Let's look at each of the elements more closely.

Step #1: Target Your Ideal Patients

After taking the action step detailed earlier in the book, you made a choice about the ideal type of patient you want to work with. You now need to move on from there and target a marketing message specifically to them.

In order to do that, you need to define who they are more clearly.

One of the ways to clearly define your ideal patient is to create an "avatar." This is just a general description of the demographic and socioeconomic characteristics of your ideal patient and is done in a way that allows you to see them as if they were an individual person rather than an anonymous mass of data.

Here's an example of the avatar that Dr. Henry created for her hormone replacement offer:

> *"Anna is a college-educated, 45-year-old female. She owns her own home and has a household annual income greater than $100,000. She is very health-conscious and follows people like Dr. Oz, Dr. Josh Axe, Dr. Mark Hyman, and Izabella Wentz on the internet.*
>
> *She is troubled by fatigue, weight gain and decreased libido. She has been to her traditional doctor with these concerns and she was told this is just a part of aging, and there is nothing really to be done about it.*
>
> *Anna is not happy with the answer she received from her traditional doctor. She thinks she may have a hormonal imbalance, so she has started to Google 'hormone replacement therapy.'"*

Keeping that avatar in mind makes it much easier for you to create advertising and marketing that speaks to your ideal patients.

With a clear target in mind, you or someone you hire can begin to write all of your marketing to speak to Anna and all the women like Anna who are looking for your services. It makes the message very personalized and it creates an attraction to you and your services.

One of our mentors, Dan Kennedy, calls this Magnetic Marketing. In this way, the selling of your services is never sleazy or salesy.

The potential client will seek you out after reading or watching some of your education-based marketing. They will ask to work with you because they see you as the authority and as someone who understands them.

Step #2: Attract Their Attention

Once you have identified your ideal patient, you need to find a way to reach out to them.

Certainly, some people will come to you through word of mouth and recommendation, but you can't solely rely on this one method of obtaining new patients.

Relying on word of mouth, particularly in a new practice, may be unpredictable and may not deliver sufficient volume to help your practice grow. Therefore, you need to have several mechanisms in place to draw people to you.

One of the most effective ways of drawing people to you is to offer them educational content in exchange for their email address.

The educational material you offer should cover a hot topic of interest for your ideal client. This information can be offered in a number of ways such as:

- Downloadable PDF report

- Email series

- Video presentation

- Checklist and resources

- Printed book

Often the easiest option is to offer a short downloadable PDF report.

For example, Dr. Woods offers a free report and a webinar on hormone balance to people who visit her website.

We'll talk more about the free report process in the next step, but clearly, it's a waste of time offering it if nobody is visiting the website.

You can't rely on people stumbling on your site or even taking the time to actively search for you.

So, you need a way to drive potential new clients to the site in order to give them the opportunity to sign up for your free offer.

There are many ways you can drive traffic to your site, but we have found that one of the most effective ways for doing this is by advertising on one of the popular social media platforms.

Personally, we have found most success with Facebook and Instagram. However, YouTube, Google and LinkedIn are all other great social media platforms that likely have hundreds of your ideal clients. We suggest starting with one social media platform and branching out from there.

This is another reason why the previous step of defining your exact ideal patient is so important. You can design ads specifically targeted to them.

You must grab their attention by speaking to their pain points. To do that, you need to think about what keeps them up in the middle of the night. What would your potential patient be searching on Google at three o'clock in the morning because they're frustrated with what's going on with their health?

In creating the advertising and the free report, you have to avoid talking in medical jargon and using technical terms. Your content needs to be more on an emotional level. People need to feel like you really get them and understand what they're going through.

You want to help them recognize their next best step is to work with you.

Here's an example of a Facebook ad that Dr. Woods uses to drive people to her website.

Feeling A Bit Off?

The most common reason why we feel terrible isn't your fault at all. It's usually because our hormones aren't functioning properly.

I'm Dr. Malaika Woods, and it's my mission to help women get back to fabulous by fighting fat and fatigue naturally.

Grab my free report, "3 Secrets of Hormones Every Woman Should Know," by clicking below. You will learn more today to start getting back on track with your hormones. Download my new report here, completely free of charge -->>

https://drwoodswellness.com/guide

You can visit www.UnlimitedHealthInstitute.com to see how Dr. Henry uses a diabetes webinar to enroll new patients.

Resource Suggestion

If you don't want to create your own free report to give away, you can hire a writer at a freelance site such as Upwork.

Step #3: Capture Their Contact Details

When someone visits your website, it's important that you try to capture their contact information.

That's why we suggest offering something like a free report or webinar as we mentioned in the previous step.

When you offer something useful and collect their contact information – at least name and email address – you can start building a relationship with them.

It's very unlikely that someone will visit your site and immediately pick up the phone to make an appointment.

While that sometimes can happen, you can't build your practice on the assumption that people will schedule with you after just one encounter.

In marketing, it is known that it takes, on average, seven different touch points before a person will make a purchase. This is relevant to all industries, even your practice.

Many people will still be in the research phase when they visit your site, and often they will need time to consider all their options before making a decision.

In the past, the technology for collecting emails was more complicated, but now there are resources available that make it all fairly straightforward.

There are a few different resources you are likely to need:

- Email system or CRM (Customer Relationship Manager) to store email addresses and send out messages. There are many systems available to do this and one that we use and like is Active Campaign.

- Sign up boxes for your website (also known as opt-ins). This can be done directly on your website e.g. using special plugins. However, there are services available that specialize in opt-ins, such as ClickFunnels and LeadPages that simplify the whole process.

- Download page for delivery of the free report. This can be on your website or on an external location, for example, if you use one of the services just mentioned.

These systems simplify the whole process of capturing email addresses and keeping in touch with your people and potential patients.

By the way, we don't recommend using your personal email account for this type of communication as it is technically more complicated and makes it difficult to ensure you comply with the legal requirements for email campaigns.

When someone goes to the download page to access their free report, we also suggest creating a short thank you video (two or three minutes) that encourages your potential patient to sign up for a strategy session.

Part of the message on the video should be, "Hey, I understand what you're going through and here's how I can help."

There is a button below the thank you video that enables them to schedule the strategy call right away using a calendar scheduling system.

While not everyone will be ready to take the next step right away, many will. So, it's important to give them that option.

Even for those who don't decide to schedule a strategy call right away, you're planting the idea in their mind that it's something they might be ready to do later.

Resource suggestions

Email and CRM system: ActiveCampaign.com, Mailchimp.com

Name capture systems: LeadPages.net, ClickFunnels.com

Appointment booking: Calendly.com, YouCanBook.me, Scheduleonce.com

Video creation: Camtasia.com

Step #4: Build Trust with Them

Capturing the contact information of your potential client is not the end goal though it is an important piece of your entire lead generation and conversion system.

Collecting the email address is not an end in its own right. You have to create a series of follow-up messages that encourage people to move forward with you.

Some people will be ready to move forward with you right away while others may need more time and information before taking the next step.

Those who are not ready right away need to receive a series of messages over time that will educate them and allow them the opportunity to get to know, like and trust you.

By staying in contact with your potential client, you will build rapport over time, and as a result, more will take the next step to work with you when the time is right. The key is you always want to be offering a next step. This could be, for example:

- Quiz

- Webinar

- Live event

- Strategy session

- Paid appointment

In the last step, we mentioned that we offer people the chance to sign up for a strategy call as soon as they download the free report. For the other examples listed above that provide more information, a strategy session is also offered.

Some people will go for that right away, but most will want to get more information before they schedule a strategy call.

One way you can offer more information is by inviting people to sign up for a free webinar or live event where you discuss in more detail common health issues impacting them daily. The webinar or live event is also a great way for people to get to know you better.

Webinars can be particularly good as you can record them once and keep using them over and over again. This is known as an "evergreen" webinar.

Live events are more time-consuming but often have a higher conversion rate. These individuals have already taken a big step to come out to see you in person and spent an hour with you, so they may be ready to make a bigger commitment.

This is also true for a webinar. Those individuals, especially if they watched it from beginning to end, may be ready to take the next step and make a small purchase.

This all depends on the person. Some people are fast action takers, and they may want to go straight to a call versus watching an hour-long webinar.

But others need more information and might prefer a webinar or a live event where they can learn more.

The key is you need to have resources and processes in place to cater to both the fast-acting and those who take more time to make a decision.

Bear in mind that building trust can take a long time, and you need a regular program of communication for people who are not ready to take the next step with you.

This may include live videos, blogs, emails, or newsletters that you send out regularly.

We generally find this type of ongoing communication needs to be at least weekly though it can be supplemented by social media communication, such as a private Facebook group.

Resource suggestion

Webinars: Zoom.us, Gotomeeting.com (Go to Webinar), Webinarjam.com

Phone consultations: Zoom.us, Ringcentral.com

Step #5. Convert Some to Patients

The ultimate aim of the whole process is to move some of the people who have given you their contact information toward making the decision to work with you.

As we highlighted in the previous step, you always want to encourage people to take the next step.

These are known as calls to action and, for example, can include:

- When someone reaches the landing page, you want them to download the free report

- At that time, you also invite them to a free strategy call

- When they download the free report, it includes another invitation to a strategy call

- As an alternative to the strategy call, you can invite them to a live event or webinar

- On the free strategy call, you can invite them to sign up for a paid consultation

- At the paid appointment, you offer them the opportunity to sign up for a program

You'll never have everyone taking the desired action at each step, so it's important to have a follow-up sequence in place based on where the prospective patient is in the process.

In some cases, you'll keep sending emails to people for years before they make a purchase. During this time, it's important to keep giving them valuable information.

Let's talk a bit more about three key steps in the process where decisions are made:

- Exposure to education-based marketing (Free report, live event, webinar)

- Strategy call

- Initial paid consultation

Exposure to your education-based marketing

The objective of education-based marketing is to motivate the potential client to take action and schedule an in-office consultation with you.

As people attend a live event, for example, they have direct exposure to you which increases the chances of them wanting to start with you now as opposed to later.

These education-based marketing strategies are a great way to reach many people at once.

For example, lots of people can download your reports, or you can get groups to join you in your office or on a webinar.

During live events and webinars, you will talk things through in more detail. Your audience will get to know you better, and because they have shown the commitment to turn up, you may have more people signing up to work with you through this method.

Again, the aim of the live event is usually to get people to come for an initial paid appointment. It is not to sell the whole program.

Strategy Call

The strategy call should generally last about 15 minutes. The objective is to find out about their problem, their concerns and whether or not they are good candidates for what you have to offer.

First of all, they should feel like they've been heard because that's something they don't often get in traditional medical practices.

You also want them to understand you have a solution for their problem.

This is not just a sales pitch. It includes finding out whether or not they can afford your services and how serious they are about moving forward to the next step.

The fact is many people are just searching for more information and are not ready to work with a trained physician who can help them.

You want to identify who's ready to take action and can step outside of the confines of insurance and invest in themselves.

You need to know how ready they are to move forward right now.

You don't want to waste your time on "tire kickers." A tire kicker is someone who goes to the car dealership, walks around the lot, kicks tires to see how sturdy they are but does not have any intention to buy a car.

There are too many people who desperately need and want your help, and that is where you need to focus your time and energy.

However, bear in mind that some people may not be ready now, or they may have friends who are your ideal clients. So, don't consider them a waste of your time! Make sure you provide some resources and information that will be helpful to them and to their friends and family.

Even in the early stages with the free strategy call, it is important to only work with those who you believe are a good fit for your program. In this way, you maximize the likelihood of success for your patient.

In our businesses, we've found that these initial calls are often best handled by one of the staff so that we can focus our time on the people who want to come in for a paid consultation.

In the early stages, you may need to do these calls yourself. It is a good way to get to know your prospective patient better and you can eventually hand over this responsibility to a staff member when the time is right.

The aim of the strategy call is to get someone to book a paid appointment. It is not to sell the program at this stage.

It's important to follow the system one step at a time. Remember, you have to "date" your prospective patient before asking for their "hand in marriage"!

You need to design the call tightly so that you can cover everything in about 15 minutes.

Initial Paid Consultation

The paid consultation is an important part of the sales process, and this is where you will offer the opportunity to join a program. This is about going into more detail to help people make the decision to work with you as they try to improve their health.

Prior to the consultation, it is important to pre-sell them on the idea of working with you. We like to send out a package in a flashy colorful bubble mailer, which includes a full-color report on one of their major health concerns.

This mailer also includes a letter stating how excited we are to meet them, a USB with patient testimonial videos and a small gift. We call this the "shock and awe" package. How many other doctors do you think have provided them with this much information and a gift prior to their first appointment? No one.

This is what we mean when we say show up like no one else. You have already made a lasting impression before they have even sat down in front of you.

The Flow of the Consultation

The consultation typically lasts about 60-90 minutes. The exact process will vary depending on the program, but here is a typical example.

- The first five or ten minutes is about building rapport and asking a few general questions to understand them better.

  We'll have a couple of minutes for greeting and ask something like, "How did you hear about us?"

  This step is to make them feel comfortable.

- The next 15 to 20 minutes is reviewing their history and identifying their major problems. We also like to ask some probing questions. We're uncovering their pain points and finding out what things are most bothersome to them. This also is a time to assess their readiness for change.

- The next 15 to 20 minutes is reviewing the labs, explaining what they mean and how it can impact their body.

We have an 18-page full color report and comprehensive lab panel. This report is highly valued and the format is powerful. It actually helps people to see their situation from another perspective.

- We then take another 15 to 20 minutes making general recommendations for them, and we write them down.

- In the last 10 to 15 minutes of the formal consultation, we explain what the program looks like. We go through the investment for the program and then answer any remaining questions.

- Then there are a few minutes at the end when we do the formal enrollment, take payment, give them their test kits, explain them and set up their next appointment.

As we've mentioned before, this is most effective when you develop scripts and presentations that you can use at various stages. You need to ensure that it flows easily when you say, "This is the investment."

During the consultation, it is important to talk about what makes you and your approach to their health concern unique.

Throughout this process, you need to address the different reasons they may be coming up with in their minds as to why they cannot purchase a program. Talk to them about stepping outside the box, investing in themselves and not having the doctor's hands tied by insurance companies.

At the conclusion of the consultation, our patients fully understand we are here to guide them through this health transformation.

Too often people view health-related issues as so bothersome and overwhelming. Therefore, we try to make the journey fun for them.

The key to a successful consultation is that your prospective patient should leave feeling it was useful whether they sign up or not. But, if you have followed the processes outlined above, most should sign up for your program.

Overview of System

The Lead Generation and Conversion System may sound quite complicated, but it's a straightforward system. Here it is in summary:

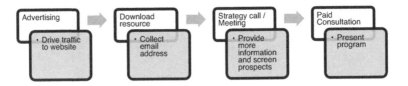

- Create an avatar of your ideal patients.

- Develop advertising and marketing that encourages them to visit your website.

- Offer them a free report or other resource in exchange for their email address.

- Aim to have as many of the people who download your report as possible attend a strategy call or live meeting.

- Aim to have a steady stream of these people attend an initial paid consultation.

- Convert as many as possible of the people who come to the paid initial consultation into paying members of your program.

- Keep in touch with the others so that more will join your program when the time is right.

Additional Systems

In addition to Lead Generation and Conversion, there are many other systems you can build into your practice to make it grow faster and run more smoothly. Here are some other systems to consider.

- **Onboarding of New Patients:** Signing people up as patients is only the start of what will hopefully be a long-term relationship and you need to get it off to the right start. You need to have a consistent and well-developed process that welcomes new patients and makes them quickly feel at home in your practice.

  For example, you can send a handwritten thank you letter that discusses how you value their commitment to health and working with you and your team. You may also choose to surprise them with a special gift, such as a gratitude journal to record their health journey.

- **Follow-up for Appointments:** You can't always rely on people to remember their scheduled appointment. Make sure your EMR (Electronic Medical Record) has built-in appointment reminders (via email and/or text message).

  You should also have a no-show policy to discourage missed appointments. When people don't show, it leads to wasted time, patients getting poor results and it costs your practice money.

- **Encouraging Referrals:** One of the most effective ways to grow your practice is through referrals from existing patients.

  However, just because you have rendered a great service, don't assume your patients will refer. You need to create a formal referral process.

  You need to ask for the referral. When you ask for the referral, make sure you explain to the patient the best way to make the introduction to the prospective patient.

Your referral system should also include a process to help your current patient feel appreciated and rewarded when they do refer others.

- **Retention and Reactivation of Patients:** In an independent practice, you can't afford to let patients go cold on you. This means do not allow them to get lost to follow-up.

  Please stay in touch with your clients either through phone calls, emails or special events just for patients. Sometimes people will have good reasons why they don't complete a program or lose touch with you. It's always your responsibility to reactivate contact when it has been lost and see if people are now ready to move forward.

- **Staff Recruitment:** As your practice grows, the recruitment of people will become more important and time-consuming. The more you can standardize and create a system around staffing recruitment, the more effective and efficient it will be.

So, while we want you to focus on Lead Generation and Conversion to get started, it's a good idea to think about what other areas of your practice would benefit from clearly defined systems.

ACTIONS

1. Develop your avatar

2. Decide on your education-based content

3. Create some follow up emails

4. Design the strategy call

5. Develop the paid initial consultation flow to promote enrollment in your full program

Chapter 9: How You Can Become the Physician Unleashed

In this book, we've covered the challenges faced by physicians in today's marketplace and we've shared the steps you need to take if you want to become the Physician Unleashed.

We started by going through some of the key reasons why so many physicians nowadays feel they are being kept on a leash – the increased pressures from administration, the power of insurance companies and the low job satisfaction.

We suggested that there are many reasons to believe that things are more likely to get worse in the future rather than better unless individual physicians take action to break free.

We hope you were inspired by the stories we shared of how we dealt with the challenges we were facing and how we were able to move forward to something better.

In the core of this book, we shared with you our Physician Freedom Formula:

$$A \times V \times S = Freedom$$

In this formula, A is Authority, V is Value and S is Systems.

The stronger you can be with each of these elements, the more success you are likely to have in breaking free.

We shared with you the five key elements of the Physician Authority Formula and gave you the outline for an action plan to make sure others know about your expertise.

We then talked about the three different elements of value and explained how you can maximize each to ensure you have very satisfied patients who pay you attractive fees and are rewarding to work with.

Finally, we talked about the importance of systems and went through in detail how to establish an effective system for lead generation and conversion.

We hope that what you've read here has not only inspired you to take action but has given you a formula that you can follow to truly break free.

We'd love to help you on this journey in any way we can. So, if you're looking to become a Physician Unleashed and would like some further help or inspiration – or you'd like to share the story of your own success – please don't hesitate to contact us at info@abundantphysician.com

Tamika Henry, MD, MBA

Malaika Woods, MD, MPH

About the Authors

- **Tamika Henry, MD, MBA** is founder and CMO of the Unlimited Health Institute in Pasadena California, where she is on a mission to eradicate fatigue, diabetes, hormonal imbalance and more from our normal lives. She always says, "Unlimited Thinking. Unlimited You!"

  For the past 13 years, she has been practicing as a board-certified family physician and she established her own independent practice in 2014.

- **Malaika Woods, MD, MPH** is principal of Dr. Woods Wellness in Lee's Summit, Missouri, where she shares her passion for empowering patients with the tools and knowledge they need to discover the root cause of their symptoms.

  Dr. Woods often shares this truth, "The human body is divinely designed and has a great capacity to heal."

  After six years as a practicing physician, she grew frustrated with the limits that large medical groups and insurance companies placed on how she could help her patients and she established her own practice in 2012.

- In addition to supporting their own patients, both Dr. Henry and Dr. Woods have a love for business. Based on what they learned in setting up their own successful practices, they established The Abundant Physician to help other doctors create the practice of their dreams. Their mission is to help physicians have a greater impact on patients' health, more personal freedom and to get paid what they're worth!

What Others Say About the Authors

"We decided to work with Dr. Henry and Dr. Woods because we were struggling with consistently having enough business income throughout the year. We also have a considerable amount of debt which limits us and which we were trying to pay down. We sought their services to help us increase income and to help us make some decisions we were considering in regards to the same.

Our experience working with Dr. Henry and Dr. Woods was great. They made themselves available to us with scheduled phone calls and emails to fill in the gaps and/or to address any interim questions or concerns we had (these were in addition to our initial in-person workshop where we developed the basis of our plan).

We found them to be wonderfully prompt in answering our questions and concerns. They gave us solid ideas as well as materials to work with. The materials were extremely helpful since we were already strapped for time and would have had a difficult time developing all the materials ourselves. One example of this was an informational/educational presentation I gave to a networking group which also promoted our services. They sent us slides as well as ideas to incorporate into the presentation.

I would definitely recommend Dr. Henry and Dr. Woods. They make a good team and between them have a breadth of experience, knowledge, and materials that can help you to increase or expand your medical practice and business – with new clients and with retaining clients – and they are fun and easy to work with!"

Delphine Shannon, M.D.
Medical Director
Health Fit M.D.
Gulfport, Mississippi

"Having the guidance of Dr. Henry and Dr. Woods has truly been invaluable. I had been considering starting a private wellness practice for some time but was reluctant because of my fears surrounding the business and logistics aspects of a private practice.

I am so grateful that I found these two dynamic physicians to mentor me. My fears have disappeared, and I am currently launching my new practice with all the confidence in the world. I know they will continue to support me along my journey. They have imparted to me the skill set to be a 'physician unleashed' and that feels amazing!"

Anne Morgan, D.O.
Medical Director
Thrive Once More
Kansas City, Missouri

Free Bonus for Readers Only

Are You Ready to Take the Next Step and Become a Profitable Abundant Physician Unleashed?

Because you invested in this book, you qualify for a chance to get a 30-Minute Freedom Formula Discovery Call. The call is designed to give you practical (and easy) ways to grow your practice, have a bigger impact, and take more time off.

On the call, we'll review your current practice (or your plans to start one) and will show you some of the areas where you can instantly create massive growth. We'll also diagnose potential gaps that are preventing you from having the practice of your dreams.

By the time we are done, you will be 100% clear on the next steps you need to take to better your lifestyle, make a bigger impact and get paid what you're worth!

To apply, visit the link below:

www.PhysicianFreedomFormula.com/discovery

Made in the USA
Coppell, TX
22 February 2021